MW00580513

FUTURE CARE

FUTURE CARE

SENSORS, ARTIFICIAL INTELLIGENCE, AND THE REINVENTION OF MEDICINE

Jag Singh

MAYO CLINIC PRESS

MAYO CLINIC PRESS
200 First St. SW
Rochester, MN 55905
mcpress.mayoclinic.org

Future Care. Copyright © 2023 by Jag Singh. All rights reserved. No part of this publication may be reproduced, stored in a retrieval system, or transmitted, in any form or by any means, electronic, mechanical, photocopying, recording, or otherwise, without the prior written permission of the publisher.

The information in this book is true and complete to the best of our knowledge. This book is intended as an informative guide for those wishing to learn more about health issues. It is not intended to replace, countermand or conflict with advice given to you by your own physician. The ultimate decision concerning your care should be made between you and your doctor. Information in this book is offered with no guarantees. The author and publisher disclaim all liability in connection with the use of this book.

The views expressed are the author's personal views, and do not necessarily reflect the policy or position of Mayo Clinic.

To stay informed about Mayo Clinic Press, please subscribe to our free e-newsletter at mcpress.mayoclinic.org or follow us on social media.

For bulk sales to employers, member groups and health-related companies, contact Mayo Clinic at SpecialSalesMayoBooks@mayo.edu.

Proceeds from the sale of every book benefit important medical research and education at Mayo Clinic.

Cover design: Pete Garceau

Library of Congress Control Number: 2022942483

ISBN: 978-1-945564-25-3

Printed in China

First edition: 2023

Dedicated to the soul of our health care system:
our nurses

CONTENTS

FOREWORD

BY SIDDHARTHA MUKHERJEE

Future Care will most certainly serve as a template for the way medical care will evolve in the coming years. I have known Jag Singh for over two decades. We both started our journey in medicine in India and completed our doctorates at Oxford (at different times); we overlapped in our training at Massachusetts General Hospital, Harvard Medical School. Jag is a doctor's doctor, a consummate clinician, tangential thinker, futurist, and scientist striving to improve the delivery of care through his research in device technologies and electrical therapies for cardiac disorders. As the former clinical lead for one of the largest cardiology divisions in the country, Jag understands the travails and tribulations of the health care system. In *Future Care*, he brings together the different evolving facets of digital health and the story of how they might interface and make health care sustainable.

Health care, as we all know, is in a state of transition. Its digital transformation using sensors and artificial intelligence will change the way we deliver and receive care. *Future Care* sits at the epicenter of public discourse about this transition. The soul of this book is centered on improving lives through forecasting and averting disease by providing well-timed interventions. Jag delivers this message with a unique simplicity and clarity, illustrated by his own personal encounters with disease and the patients in his care. The book is vibrantly punctuated with real-life clinical situations, with scores of stories, anecdotes, and characters. I was particularly struck by Victoria's story (her seven family members are dying of cancer, and she seeks an understanding of how to care for them) and by Maya, a 38-year-old woman losing her battle with pancreatic cancer and struggling to come to terms with her mortality. These narratives highlight several areas where transformative technologies—including artificial intelligence to aid in the early detection, or guide the treatment, of cancer—can help save lives. The memorable story of Laura and her failing heart and devastating collapse emphasizes how much angst could so easily be prevented through the remote monitoring of sensor data.

The burgeoning digital metamorphosis in medicine provides us an opportunity to scale personalized care globally. To that end, this book highlights new models of care and provides a vision for what the hospital of the future might look like. Importantly, none of this seems dystopian. Jag has very comprehensively outlined the need for modular medicine, disease management models, and third-party vendors, while postulating the evolution of the classic academic medical center. Some of this digital transformation is already here; it has just not yet found its way into clinical practice. We have a unique opportunity to understand and embrace this new world of sensors and artificial intelligence—and adapt it to our lives.

Future Care will have a significant impact on how medicine continues to evolve. It will serve as a terrific guide for patients, caregivers, and anyone interested in health care as it provides direction for the future.

FUTURE CARE

PROLOGUE

Sunlight streaming through the large, uncovered windows woke me. I opened my eyes to a room I had come to know intimately. I was in a hospital bed. There were graying wooden cabinets and a boxy TV in front of me, windows to my left, and a lone faded sofa facing the bed in which I now spent nearly the entirety of my time. Flanking me were two steel IV poles: one with a mounted iPad that facilitated communication with the nurses and the other holding my medications and IV fluids. If I craned my neck to look behind me, I could glimpse the monitor displaying my heart rate, oxygen saturation levels, and blood pressure. This was what I had begun to call home. It was early March 2020. The pandemic was still new—something made painfully obvious by the fact that no one really knew what to do. There were no approved medicines yet. There was no clear set of treatment guidelines. There was little from the past with which to create a care pathway. What we had in spades was speculation.

My COVID-19 journey began in the emergency room, where my dipping oxygen saturations and ghastly chest X-ray and CT scans saw me immediately transferred to the intensive care unit. The hospital staff was preparing for possible ventilator support, but my oxygen levels stayed stable enough that I was able to be moved from the intensive care unit to the COVID floor of the hospital. The doctors had told me that I would lose my sense of smell, but that wasn't an accurate description of what I experienced. Instead of not being able to smell what was in front of me, I was overwhelmed by a putrid, pungent odor. For every second of the day, the smell—and taste—assaulted me. I felt constantly reminded that the virus had stationed itself in my nasopharynx. It was now commandeering my body.

During my time in the hospital, I was racked with fever, and a deep ache settled throughout my entire body. I could see the toll the sickness was taking on me every time I looked in the mirror. I had lost nearly fifteen pounds, and my clothes hung loosely around my frame. My cough lingered, and my oxygen levels hovered at a level that had me continually anxious I'd be put on oxygen support. The oxygen saturation monitor clipped onto my finger usually displayed figures in the low nineties. When it occasionally dipped into the eighties, I would take breaths as deep as I was able and try to drag myself out of bed to expand my lungs. I didn't want the nurse to notice the low numbers, as I had no interest in going back to the ICU.

My medical background enabled me to assess the situation with some clarity. I had widespread pneumonia involving both lungs. I knew that any downward trend in my oxygen saturation levels meant the virus was winning the fight. At fifty-five years old, I had come to terms with the possibility of an unfavorable outcome. Terrible reports were drifting in from France and Italy about the difficulty of weaning patients off ventilators and the subsequent premature deaths that occurred. I was grateful my stay in the ICU had been brief and that I had escaped the need for a mechanical ventilator, but I still knew I was not doing well.

And that frustrated me. I just couldn't figure it out. I had always been healthy, aside from diabetes that I controlled through diet and exercise. I had never once been hospitalized. I had not missed a single day of work over my three decades of looking after patients. It wasn't that I was surprised to have contracted COVID; as a physician, I considered it an occupational hazard. I knew the virus seemed to be agnostic to demographics or prior good health, so falling victim myself seemed fair enough. What I was shaken by was the rapid downturn of events that necessitated my hospitalization. I figured I'd do pretty well if I contracted the virus, but I most certainly was not. At that time when I felt so low, I was intensely grateful for my family and for the technology that allowed us to communicate face-to-face even as visitors were barred from my room. They were there to encourage me and remind me of their love several times a day. While I am generally not a sentimental person, I felt vulnerable and in need of emotional bolstering. In video calls with my family, I often found myself unable to respond with anything more than a single word or a shake of my head, lest my voice crack and expose the depth of my helplessness. It wasn't unusual for me to abruptly hang up, on the verge of tears. But it was so good to see their faces nonetheless, and their calls helped me focus on getting better.

The longest walk I could manage was the six steps to the bathroom, which left me gasping for breath with an air-hunger I had never experienced. The only comparison I've come up with that seems to accurately illustrate the desperation I felt to fill my lungs would be if someone attempted to breathe through a straw while sprinting. The struggle to breathe in the face of such minimal exertion was disconcerting, to say the least. My cough and fluctuating temperature ate away at my reserves. I had quickly lost much of my muscle mass and was startled to find I could encircle my upper thigh with my two hands. I felt most comfortable lying in bed. The fear of being sent back to the ICU lingered. I knew it could happen quickly, as I had already signed the consent form agreeing to emergent intubation, mechanical ventilator support, and invasive hemodynamic lines if the supervising clinicians deemed them necessary. Despite my physical exhaustion, I was determined to do my bit by carrying out the lung exercises my nurse had shown me using the incentive spirometer left by my bedside. I was meant to exhale deeply into the instrument, but often had to stop because of my cough.

One of the few distractions from my own discomfort was the sound of distant coughing emanating from elsewhere on the COVID floor. I found I was able to chart the worsening condition of my closest neighbors based on the noises they made and the subsequent hubbub of activity in the corridor outside their rooms when the situations came to a head. When I felt bold enough, I'd ask after them, only to be told the unfortunate neighbor was now in the ICU in respiratory distress, needing to be intubated and put on a ventilator.

It was lonely. Not only was I isolated from family and kept separate from the other patients on the floor, but the staff who came in to take my vitals were understandably masked and gowned, depriving me of the human connection I so craved. I wasn't even sure if the same nurses were helping me every day. I didn't think I'd be able to recognize a single person who came into my room at that time in any other context—if I made it out alive, that was. Yet despite its clear limitations, I was deeply appreciative of any human interaction. Visits from my physicians and nurses were the only nondigital face-to-face time I had with anyone, as brief and fabric cloaked as they were. But as the days passed, the visits became shorter and more infrequent before giving way fully to video calls. The iPad strapped to the IV pole on the left side of my bed would beep on, and I'd know it was time for a quick virtual check-in. It seemed that even in-hospital care was somehow becoming remote care. At first, I was jarred. But bedridden as I was, I had time to consider. Video visits kept health care providers from unnecessary exposure to a patient who could be actively shedding the virus. And really, there wasn't much to do or treat—the care my medical team provided was all palliative. We were waiting to see who would win: the virus or the human.

For the first seven days on the COVID floor, my readings looked grim. But on the eighth day, when the iPad beeped on, the doctor was smiling into the camera. My blood tests looked good, she said. The concerning markers we had been most worried about had begun to downtrend. The doctor told me she had reviewed my heart rate, blood pressure, temperature, and oxygen saturations from the display on the monitor outside my room. She thought it was time for me to go home. The hospital was filling up with more COVID patients, she said, and they were running short on beds.

Perhaps sensing my disorientation at such a sudden about-face regarding my condition, the doctor assured me that my vital signs and clinical course could easily be evaluated remotely. Recent advancements in telemedicine meant I could be efficiently and effectively treated from home. She talked me through the tools and sensors I'd be using to measure my temperature, blood pressure, heart rate, and oxygen saturations from the comfort of my own bedroom. My head spun. While I had been ill for more than three weeks, it was still very early in the pandemic—yet even over the short time I'd been confined to my hospital bed, I had watched the infrastructure for and reliance upon virtual care progress at a dizzying rate. Even then it seemed clear: the shift may have been born of necessity, but it was here to stay.

INTRODUCTION

The future of health care will be virtual, aided by sensor strategies and powered by predictive analytics. This will enable personalized decisions and, consequently, the delivery of the highest level of patient-centric care. Attentive care will be wherever the patient is and will be provided whenever the patient desires. Over the course of the next decade, this is the direction in which the practice of medicine will evolve. The transition will be tough, but we will all learn to adapt, and it may ultimately be for the better.

Health care is a multifaceted and highly complex industry. Its daily operations intersect incessantly with rapidly progressive science, unstable markets, transient fads, extravagant marketing, and unpredictable human behavior. The yin and yang of these influences result in endless conflict, contradictions, and often chaos. One of the biggest impediments to the digital transformation of care delivery has been the inertia and discomfiture inherent in sidestepping the status quo that both patients and providers are used to. The pandemic forced us all to step out of our comfort zones into a world of masks and social distancing. Self-preservation, coupled with the need to provide and receive care, catalyzed the adoption of virtual strategies. And now we have sensors that can be implanted within the human body or embedded in a slew of wearables, such as watches, earpieces, necklaces, rings, bracelets, bodysuits, belts, socks, shoes, and diapers—with the first generation of sensors that monitor heart rate being ubiquitous. This in turn has created an opportunity for these sensors to remotely provide objective data on the disease state and organ function, ensuring that a virtual video visit could be a suitable replacement for in-person interaction.

The reality is, like most features of modern life, human organs are being digitized. Sensors are well on their way to helping us proactively capture the information needed to predict and prevent disease. Medical care that has heretofore been periodic and transactional will soon become continuous. Paired with the medical world's growing emphasis on wellness and prevention, the digital revolution will help to effectively address chronic diseases that have been the health care system's Achilles' heel. This large-scale transition not only will reshape the patient-physician relationship but also will dramatically change how hospitals and the business of medicine operate. To fully benefit from the shift, however, we need to adapt not only in how we function as clinicians and patients but also in how we structure the accompanying financial and organizational workflow integration. The goal is for health care to become as sensible, affordable, and practical as possible.

It's a brave new world, and sensors are everywhere. There is a race on within the world of start-ups to find and fine-tune the best array of sensors that can interface with our electronic health records. Hospital systems are creating not just command stations to monitor hospital flow and efficiency but also sensor-driven approaches to managing and treating patients on a beat-to-beat basis. This means continuous monitoring of every individual with an electronic medical record. The provision of steady streaming of this anonymized digital data will enable us to predict and prevent flare-ups and, possibly, disease itself. Gone are the days of being reactive; this is the era of proactive care. This book uses real-life examples to detail how the ever-expanding reach of digital health, through an amalgam of virtual visits and sensor-based approaches fueled with artificial intelligence, will morph the way we experience medicine.

As a cardiac electrophysiologist, I have spent the past two decades of my life dealing with patients who have survived sudden cardiac arrests, have heart failure with life-threatening arrhythmias, live with a spectrum of annoying heart-rhythm disturbances such as atrial fibrillation (A-fib) and extra heartbeats, and others who remain highly vulnerable to dying suddenly from a variety of genetic or environmental factors. I have spent many hours either implanting pacemakers and defibrillators or burning and freezing critical electrical circuits within the hearts of thousands of my patients. Over this period, I have been engaged in research that has included basic science, epidemiology, clinical trials, and medical innovation. Much of this research has focused on developing patient-centric efforts to improve clinical outcomes and prevent sudden death while alleviating the burdensome symptoms from heart-rhythm disorders. More than ten years ago, my team and I developed one of the first sensor-derived risk scores to help stratify and predict poor clinical outcomes and mortality in our heart failure patients with data collected from sensors in the pacemakers and defibrillators implanted in the chests and hearts of many patients. Simple measures of physical activity, nocturnal heart rate, and autonomic activity could tell us which patients had a fivefold increased risk of dying within one year. More recently, I have researched and validated sophisticated integrated sensor strategies that have a higher predictive value and a higher specificity in predicting life-altering occurrences such as heart failure exacerbations, malignant heart-rhythm events, hospitalizations, and death. The identification of a subgroup of high-risk patients enables proactive interventions to improve their quality and quantity of life, which, frankly, is the holy grail of medicine.

I have also used deep neural networks and machine learning to predict sickness and potentially shift in-hospital care to the home. Within the next decade, we will have organized data streams that will allow us to simulate the clinical course of patients through the construct of an avatar-like digital double. Creating a digital twin of the real-world patient using multiple sensors will provide us with the means to forecast health problems and proactively intervene, oftentimes remotely. Digitizing ourselves will help us move from analyzing the past to predicting the future. This will obviously require quadrillions of data points, hundreds of data scientists, and service teams that focus on the bigger picture beyond immediate health issues. We will need to pay attention to the comprehensive longitudinal view of the patient journey. This is where implementation of preventative strategies will help shrink costs with value-based revenue models that promote self-management and make patients partly responsible for their own health.

This book is divided into four main parts. The first explains the origin and evolution of sensors, including an exploration of the different types available and examples of their use through real patient stories, as well as a forecast of what they soon will be capable of. The second covers the nuances of telehealth and its impact on access to care and delivery, acknowledging the effect the digital revolution has had on patient experience, the deepening divide of social disparities, and a host of other equally pressing issues. The third deals with artificial intelligence (AI), beginning with a primer on what AI is before taking a deep dive into the building tsunami of data, its impact, and its clinical applicability, along with the ethical aspects and biases we must consider as part of the conversation. The last part anchors the revelations of the first three into the context of the current health care landscape, with a focus on the principles that make a health care system sustainable. That section also examines the impact of COVID on our future, changing reimbursement models, and the participation of the patient in their own care. The book concludes with a vision for what the hospital of the future might look like—a vision tethered to the practical and realistic, rather than one that indulges the grandiose or dystopian.

Much of the discourse in this book aims to empower the reader in recognizing this future and thereby playing a part in how it all unfolds. The intent here is to be realistic about the hurdles, while compelling regulatory bodies and the payers to recognize the direction of the blowing wind so they can adjust their sails. The positive impacts on patient experience, costs, and clinical outcomes will vanquish barriers and allow care to cross state and national borders.

Change is inevitable. The intersection of the world of sensors with virtual care and AI-based algorithms will demand change for the next several years. More sensors mean more data; more data means more resources to store, analyze, and generate algorithms; more algorithms and more data could mean less privacy, so it may not all turn out to be hunky-dory. The downstream impact on care patterns, workflow, job descriptions, hospital economics, privacy, and the overall geopolitics of health care are unpredictable. This book focuses on addressing these issues, especially the need to modernize our workflows and redeploy and repurpose many of the current clinical roles, while making health care more accessible, equitable, and accountable.

At the same time, established academic medical centers are morphing and trying to redefine themselves. Many clinicians are leaving conventional hospital practice to begin start-ups that focus on the delivery of personalized primary care and disease management programs. Deep structural changes that depart from the conventional care-delivery architecture are falling into place. New technologies and AI assets will engender new workflows that transcend the boundaries of primary and specialty care. The academic center of the future will be one that provides tertiary- and quaternary-level care across state and national borders and focuses on rare and complex diseases while working with local third-party vendors to provide primary care. Whether you are an interested reader, technologist, patient, physician, nurse, advanced care practitioner, hospital administrator, or business leader, this book will provide you with some insight into the future digital transformation of health care. It will deliberate the change in the practice of medicine and the evolving reimbursement schemes that will make it sustainable. For the financial analyst or a venture capitalist, this will provide a structure for developing investment models and decisions. This book will postulate the framework for this change, while paying attention to each of the trade-offs.

My aim is for readers to be empowered through their growing understanding of the short- and long-term strategies for promoting wellness, treating chronic ailments, or improving outcomes from common but devastating illnesses such as cancer, diabetes, heart disease, kidney failure, lung problems, COVID-19, and so on. I firmly believe that a better understanding of the newly developing health care pathways and their many intricacies will become increasingly crucial as society acclimates to the morphing landscape. The technology is already here; now we must understand it, adapt to it, and embrace it.

OUR BIG, FAT, SICK HEALTH CARE SYSTEM: THE NEED FOR CHANGE

Change is not merely necessary to life—it is life.
ALVIN TOFFLER

As much as we may like to think the US is the most powerful nation with the best health system, we know this is far from the truth. Our system is plagued with millions of uninsured patients, inexplicable costs for routine care, high levels of patient dissatisfaction, and distressingly low life expectancies. The latter are among the lowest in the developed world. The current system is indefensible on both cost-effectiveness and quality of care.

Add to this the unpredictable access, discrepancies between rural and urban regions, and disparities in medical care when stratified by socioeconomic status and race, and we have a mess on our hands. The drain on the national treasury is so colossal that delivering health care in its current form has had a destructive bearing on other areas of community services, resources, and consequently innovation. It behooves us to think holistically about trying to fix this situation—not through singular, independent efforts, but through collaborative ones that can help give us the health care we deserve.

There are many reasons for our fat and sick health care system. If I were to generalize, I would say a big part of this corpulence ensues from the unconscionable self-indulgence of pharmaceutical establishments, insurance companies, health care executives, and hospital systems. Another part is a consequence of the inefficiencies in the administration of health care, due to duplicative efforts, archaic managerial routines, and a lack of uniform streamlined processes at both the front and back ends of care delivery. It may not come as a surprise that more than a quarter of the costs of health care are generated by middle managers and the absence of standardized procedures within and between hospital systems. The nationwide deployment of electronic medical records (EMRs) has helped, but it is mind-boggling to see the variability in practice, including scheduling, answering patient calls, pre-authorizations, medical record coding, and claims submission. Consequently, the waste is astounding.

When it comes to self-indulgence, sometimes it's difficult to discern where this occurs. We know about Pharma hiking the prices of new drugs and taking advantage of vulnerable patients and institutions. Rebate swindles remain common, with good deals for favored hospitals and higher prices for nonpreferred ones. Costs for most drugs, devices, and procedures are several times higher in the US than in other countries. Hospitals are to blame here, too. We know for certain that renowned hospitals charge prices multiple times higher than those at lesser-known institutions. Even though this may be considered partially acceptable for complex procedures and surgeries, it certainly doesn't seem appropriate for routine tests, such as electrocardiograms (ECGs) and chest X-rays. In hospitals across the US, the cost of an X-ray can vary from $41 to a high of nearly $300, while a head computed tomography (CT) scan can vary from $100 to more than $2,000. It is mind-blowing that the same implantable device, such as a defibrillator, can cost under $10,000 at a leading academic center, $35,000 at a small community hospital, but $3,000 in Europe or even less in India. Almost the same discrepancy exists for other imaging and diagnostic tests all across the US.

THE CHANGING PLAYING FIELD

It is quite remarkable when one looks at the rank order of the largest US companies in 2008 compared to 2020. In 2008, only one tech company—Microsoft, ranked number three—was in the top five. In 2020, the top five companies—Apple, Google, Microsoft, Amazon, and Facebook—were all tech companies, and each of them was focused on disrupting health care. It is inevitable that the way we dispense care is going to change, and much of it may be dictated by these giant high-tech companies, as well as their partnerships, mergers, and acquisitions, which already play a significant role in shaping market forces and dynamics. Hospital systems are doing the same to stay relevant and scaling up their cloud-computing capabilities. As an example, Kaiser Permanente is in a deal with Microsoft and Accenture to support the digital experience of more than twelve million members and nearly ninety thousand clinicians.

Cynically, we may look at this partnership as nonaltruistic and an attempt to gain access to a multibillion-dollar market and generate profits for shareholders; however, one cannot help conceding that this is a worthy venture, if the collateral benefit is that it will make health care more efficient and cost-effective. Other new partnerships include giants CVS Health and Aetna, Cigna and Express Scripts, Humana and Kindred Healthcare, and the Walmart-Humana merger. All of them are motivated toward uprooting the conventional current models of health care delivery. The recent Teladoc takeover of Livongo, which provides diabetes monitoring and remote monitoring, speaks for itself. The combination of two of the largest publicly traded virtual care companies will create a health technology goliath (worth $37 billion) just as the need for virtual care increases exponentially. Walgreens recently opened between five hundred and one thousand doctor offices, with a provision of round-the-clock care, either in person or virtually, with pharmacists and doctors working jointly. The alliance with VillageMD will allow Walgreens to staff these offices with more than three thousand primary care physicians (PCP). This will enhance access and provision of care to patients with chronic disease, allowing frequent evaluations, monitoring, and medication adjustments—much of this usefully located in a convenience store. The giant digital companies (e.g., Google and Amazon) are crafting a widely used accessible virtual infrastructure that may redefine what the market should look like. These companies have an extensively available cloud-based system that could provide a service, but how this integrates within the hospital financial model is unclear. Will this lead to a fee per patient or fee per service, and will it be paid for by the patient, insurance, or hospital practice? One of the top challenges inherent in health care is the need to provide patient-centric, personalized care but at the population level and in a uniform way.

The biggest disruption on how health care will drive the market (or vice versa) will be determined by the wizardry of technology and its adoption. High-tech companies are betting on the combination of the increase in computing power and the availability of large datasets to change the face of the delivery of medical and surgical care. For sure, this will change the norms of patient-physician interactions and raise the bar for health care, which AI can and will transform. The pre-COVID–era projections suggested that AI will help save the health care economy $150 billion by 2026. As the pandemic settles, subsequent projections may be much higher. Goldman Sachs estimates that digitizing many parts of the working apparatus of health care could result in savings exceeding $300 billion. More than two-thirds of these savings will come from management of chronic diseases, especially because much of the care for those conditions could be sensor-aided and remote.

COST AND CARE

Noticeably, the big attraction remains that health care continues to grow at a fast clip—almost double the rate of other industries. Approximately one-fifth of the gross domestic product comes from health care, which totals nearly $4 trillion a year and is manyfold higher than the economy of several well-to-do European nations. Pre-pandemic, the compounded annual growth rate for the US health care sector was projected to increase by 5 to 7 percent, to as high as approximately $670 billion. COVID-19 and its aftermath shattered some of the euphoria, leaving hospitals facing huge increases in costs. Much of this stems from labor and medical supply expenses, each having increased by approximately 20 percent, causing one-third of hospitals to run at a negative margin.

We have a sick system. Beyond this actual cost, the utilization of services (especially of imaging and high-end technology) is another big contributor to the astronomical spending. Pursuing margins and treatments that reimburse well, rather than prioritizing preventative approaches to disease, has contributed to this systemic illness. A part of the disconnect is that hospitals and insurance companies are looking down at their feet, hoping not to stumble and fall. There is no front-facing vision paying attention to the entire human life cycle and lifetime. Our approach to care is transactional and transient, yearly from budget to budget, one-year term insurance policies, while diseases have lifelong spending implications. There is no accountability or incentive within the system to prioritize health and prevention of illnesses. The American health care system is opaque, inefficient, inept, and inequitable. It is gravely sick and in need of resuscitation.

It is time to lift the linen, see what's below, and share it. Understanding the dysfunctional elements of modern-day American medicine and then choosing methods to sort through them using digital technology will allow us to pick away at each one of them. Even though digital strategies have invaded all forms of daily living, such as ordering stuff on Amazon, hailing cars, booking hotels, dining, and banking, the one industry that has continued to drag its feet and stay aloof is health care. Most likely, it is the complexity of the many interactions and that human life is at stake that have contributed to the slow takeover.

This is where COVID-19 came to the rescue. Paradoxically, the virus infected the system with an unforeseen energy to resurrect itself—or at least it has given us that opportunity. It is truly inane that it takes a pandemic or a national disaster to get us out of our state of inertia. But that opportunity seems to be our silver lining. Telehealth and virtual care allowed for the practice of medicine and the care of patients in their homes. The pandemic has reset patient expectations of care, which has the governments and regulators desperately trying to codify some of the changes that have worked so well.

TIME FOR TRANSITIONS

The takeover is imminent, and the transition has begun. We need to rebuild from ground zero. Enhancing transparency and accountability, redefining our value proposition, and restructuring our institutions is the only way forward. The conversation around data, health, wearables, sensors, and AI is now center stage. Even before all this, there was evidence that the winds of change were here. Market trends had already begun making health care organizations examine how we practice medicine, necessitating that we become nimbler and more patient-centric, and improve outcomes—at lower costs. In 2020, approximately 80 percent of health care expenses went toward treatment, and it is expected that by 2040, 60 percent of spending will go toward health, wellness, and disease prevention, bringing down health care spending in its totality.

As we plan for these shifts in care, it is important to remember that over the coming years there will be a shortage of subspecialists and a shift in the demographic profile of our patients. Currently, there are fifty million Americans over the age of sixty-five, and it is projected that this number will double to one hundred million by 2060. Senior citizens will comprise 25 percent of the population. This tsunami of sicker and older patients could overwhelm the health care system. Add to this an aging workforce, and we have a problem. In a few years, the Gen Xers and millennials will be caregivers to the baby boomers—different generations with different expectations.

The "skipped-generation effect" will be in play here. The generation at maximal risk handles or adapts to technology differently than the one providing the care. The older strata in the baby-boomer patient population may be averse to high-tech or computer-based approaches for consultations, versus the millennials providing the care, who have cozied up to the concept of less in-person and more virtual contact. Even older practicing physicians are unenthusiastic about learning this new patient-physician interaction. Care pathways for folks of different demographics, literacy, and preferences will evolve. Compromises will be made, and cultural barriers to remote care and sensor-based approaches will steadily disappear. It is time for these transitions. I believe that virtual care strategies aided by sensors and artificial intelligence coupled with self-management approaches will create the sustainable disruption we seek and appropriate reimbursement models we need.

PART I

SENSORS

1

MAKING SENSE OF SENSORS

All our knowledge begins with the senses.
IMMANUEL KANT

I met Anil on an evening in late May 1988, when I was scheduled for a night shift in the intensive care unit at David Sassoon General Hospital in Pune, India. Anil was in his early twenties and had just been moved to the ICU because he was unable to breathe on his own and needed to be emergently intubated and receive ventilator support. He was an engineering student in the throes of preparing for his exams. About ten days earlier, he had caught a stomach bug, from which he'd since recovered, but over the past four days, he had begun to experience tingling and numbness in his legs and hands, accompanied by increasing difficulty in getting out of bed. Even raising his hands was painful and nearly impossible. He was not only unable to grasp a coffee mug but could not even feel it. Over the next twenty-four hours, all this worsened, and by the time he got to the hospital, he was having difficulty breathing.

I remember that night in the ICU particularly well because there was a power failure. Recurrent breakdowns of the electric grid were not uncommon at that time, and we were equipped with a backup generator that could kick in to support our small inventory of four very basic ventilators. That night the generator failed, and we took turns manually ventilating three patients in the ICU with the Ambu Bag, a self-inflating bag that one must rhythmically squeeze to provide positive pressure ventilation to a patient who is unable to breathe. We were short-staffed that night and I took the onus for Anil's care, squeezing one breath every five to six seconds for the next four hours or so, into the wee hours of the morning. Much of that night it remained unclear to me why Anil had deteriorated so rapidly, with paralysis of all four limbs and breathing muscles. I prayed with each squeeze that this would be reversible.

Early that morning, Dr. R. S. Wadia, legendary neurologist and role model for many aspiring doctors, walked into the ICU with an entourage of resident doctors, spoke quietly with Anil's mother to get some insight into the progression of Anil's symptoms, then performed a detailed neurological exam. In a matter of minutes, he made the diagnosis of Guillain-Barré syndrome. He wrote some illegible notes in the chart, recommended intravenous steroids, reassured the family, and left.

Guillain-Barré syndrome is a rapidly progressing condition where the body's immune system attacks the peripheral nerves that control muscle movement, as well as those nerves that transmit sensations of touch, temperature, and pain. It can also affect the entire network of cranial nerves and central nervous system, cause respiratory paralysis, limit eye movement and vision, and make it impossible to swallow. It can affect the entire neural network within the body and the accompanying senses that we all take for granted. Anil got better over the next few days. The paralysis and neural involvement began to recede, and he was able to breathe on his own again. The ventilator was disconnected a week later, and he slowly began to regain some strength and sensations in his hands and legs. He was discharged after another two weeks to begin a journey of recovery that could take several more months.

Even in the early days of my medical school training, I had been fascinated by the clinical exam of the nervous system. Through a detailed history extricated from the patient, complemented by an extensive checklist of clinical tests and maneuvers, one was able to crudely evaluate the complexity of the cerebral cortex and its seamless integration with the neural highway connecting the entire body and its organs in a swath of nerves. This involved a meticulous exam assessing attention, memory, and cognition, and tests to ensure the normal function of the cerebellum and neural tracts along with a comprehensive evaluation of the motor and sensory system. A clinical exam assessing the movement of the extremities with or without applying counter-resistance enabled the examiner to gauge the strength of each of the muscle groups in all four limbs. I watched Dr. Wadia tap at Anil's elbow, knee, and ankle joints with a rubber-nosed hammer to elicit neural tendon reflexes, which provided an overview of the intact innervation of the individual muscles.

It was, however, the sensory exam that totally mesmerized me. Testing the sensory nervous system served to remind me of the complexity of the innervation of our bodies and the simple senses that we take for granted. Testing for the sensations of touch, temperature, and pain across all quadrants of the body was performed with the touch of the hand, a wisp of cotton, a test tube holding hot or cold water, a pin, or whatever else you had handy, such as the end of a pencil or pen. Examining the cranial nerves and testing for the higher senses of smell, taste, sight, sound, and proprioception using light, smelling salts, or vibrating tuning forks never failed to remind me that there is so much here that does not meet the eye. The interlacing of our senses with our sophisticated higher intelligence, all a conglomeration of electrical impulses flowing through synaptic connections, was a reminder of the magnificence of our humanness. Our understanding, or lack thereof, behind the stimulus to test the senses and the sophistication of the neural pathways and electric circuitry within the brain is beyond humbling. Our ability to assess all these highly specialized neural functions is flawed, imperfect, and primitive. But what if we could have a way of at least measuring these neural connections more accurately and continuously?

Our bodies are an intricately connected crisscross of sensors. The entire human frame is interlaced with a network of sensory nerves running between the brain and every organ, tissue, and cell. The sensory system is a web of dendritic projections extending from the receptors on single cells, serving as a highway for coded electrical information through a maze of sensory neurons, ganglia, and neural pathways. As Alessandro Benedetti stated in 1497, "By means of nerves, the pathways of the senses are distributed like the roots and fibers of a tree."

Highly specialized groups of cells, or molecular receptors, serve as sensors to the outer world, transducing external sensory stimuli enabling vision, hearing, touch, taste, smell, and balance. These stimuli travel through the sensorineural network to the command center, our brain, which decodes these signals, permitting our awareness of the world around us. This sensory system is not unique to humans, but in fact exists in all life-forms, with a varied emphasis on the development of the senses. The extent to which the senses evolve depends on the evolution of that particular species, helping humans and other animals alike adapt to the environment while ensuring their survival.

We know that within some forms of wildlife, there is a heightened sense of smell and vision to enable the appropriate response to sustenance and threats. Some animals sense the world in ways that are beyond human perception. For example, some are able to sense electrical and magnetic fields. Interestingly, magnetoreception, the ability to align oneself with the earth's magnetic field, seems to be a trait to help birds with migration and also has been observed in bees and cattle. This is not something we humans can do very well without the aid of a compass. The duck-billed platypus has a highly developed sensor that can locate its prey through electroreception, which involves the detection of electrical impulses from its prey through sensors in its bill. And bats use sound (echolocation) to navigate their flight, find their way in the dark, and locate food.

OUR SENSES

Basically, there are five traditional human senses: hearing, sight, smell, touch, and taste. Some form of stimulation is required to perturb the receptors (sensors) and activate these senses. Depending on the type, location, intensity, and duration of the stimuli, there are receptors that are set to respond, sending the information to the brain, where it is processed to generate the appropriate response. The nerves bringing the signals from the receptors to the cerebral cortex are called the afferent nerves, while those bringing back the response are the efferent nerves. As an example, touch or pain (sharp or blunt) can stimulate the mechanoreceptors on the skin or hand. This then is interpreted at the cortical level, and the decision to respond is transmitted back. Simply put, a sensor (receptor) with an afferent connection going to the brain and an efferent limb of that circuit coming back to elicit a response constitutes the backbone of all sensor-based strategies.

It is a physical stimulus that excites the appropriate receptor to initialize the sensory experience. These receptors are widely distributed across the body, serving different functions. Mechanoreceptors feel touch, pressure, or pain; chemoreceptors are stimulated by a chemical stimulus, such as change in oxygen saturation, electrolytes, pH, lactate levels, and so on; thermoreceptors are stirred by temperature; and photoreceptors in the eyes are excited by light. The fundamental process involves the conversion of the stimulus into an electrical action potential that then finds its way up the afferent electrical axis all the way to the cerebral cortex to be processed, interpreted, and responded to.

Our senses of touch and temperature allow humans to steer away from extremes of environmental challenges and preserve ourselves from injury. Just recently, in 2021, Drs. David Julius and Ardem Patapoutian received the Nobel Prize in Physiology or Medicine for their discovery of molecular receptors for temperature and mechanical force. These mechanosensitive receptors are largely within the skin and musculoskeletal systems and recognize a variety of human sensory experiences ranging from touch to the stretch of a full bladder. These same receptors can drive many sensations, including pleasure, pain, and discomfort. The stimuli are different and the neural pathways distinctive. But the principles of the underlying reflex arc remain the same.

Smell and taste are generated by "chemo-sensors" within the olfactory or gustatory system respectively, triggered by a chemical stimulus. For example, odorant molecules (e.g., the smell of coffee, roses, or perfumes) bind to the olfactory receptor neurons in the nasal cavity, setting off the cerebral circuit of recognition and response. The complexity of the sense of vision is mind-boggling and reflective of nature's highest level of sophistication. Sight is our ability to perceive visible light and generate images on the photoreceptors in the retina, which generate electrical impulses of different patterns, hues, colors, and brightness. Any attempt to break down the chemical reactions to explain something that works almost flawlessly every second of our daily existence seems inadequate. The sensors for vision are three main types of receptors: rods, cones, and ganglion cells. Rods are photoreceptors that are sensitive to the intensity of light, cones respond to color, and the ganglion cells reside in the retina and are involved in the central nervous system autonomic response. Rods allow for vision in dim light, and the ratio of rods to cones is in some way a determinant or a correlate of which animals are diurnal or nocturnal. Of the more than one million ganglion cells in the retina, a small percentage do not contribute to vision but are photosensitive and may be involved in the acceleration of our heart rate and elevation of our blood pressure the moment we open our eyes from being asleep. Interestingly, the higher incidence of heart attacks and sudden death notable in humans in the morning hours has been attributed to this early-morning eye-opening sympathetic reflex.

Hearing, a sense for sound perception, occurs through the stimulation of the hair cells (similar to guitar strings) within the inner ears by sound vibrations. These vibrations are mechanically conducted through the eardrum and generate electrical nerve impulses that are transmitted through the auditory nerve all the way to the auditory section of the cerebral cortex. Akin to this, taste is generated by the sensors within the taste buds on the upper surface of the tongue. Thermoreceptors respond to temperature change, with two distinct types of sensory receptors for heat and cold. And then there are the nociceptors, which respond to pain or nociceptive stimuli of heat, cold, or excessive pressure that are rapidly processed by the brain and result in an immediate adaptive response, such as withdrawal. The primary motive of pain is to alert us to danger and aid us in avoiding it. Beyond these, we possess a variety of other senses—a kinesthetic sense, also known as proprioception, and balance, along with assorted other internal stimuli, such as a sense of hunger or thirst. Another distinct sense is that of sexual stimulation, which involves an interplay of several sensibilities and is tied to an array of chemical triggers and hormonal stimuli.

These peripheral sensors send signals to the sensory cortex within the brain. The central command region for each sense is distinct, with the sensory cortex including the somatosensory, visual, auditory, olfactory, or gustatory cortices. Each of these areas has separate representation within the brain and is responsible for processing the afferent signals (i.e., stimulus) and dispensing the efferent signals for instituting the appropriate response. All the information is integrated in the association cortex, enabling higher-level neural processing. Intriguingly, our very own sensory system provides us with a road map for the future of care delivery.

The hospital command center of the future is analogous to the association cortex, while the different senses and their respective representation in the brain are reflective of the different service areas within the walls of the hospital. (See Part IV, Chapter 18.) Each service area receives sensory input that is processed and sent on to the command center, where the information is desegregated, enabling the delivery of integrated personalized care.

THE ANALOG-DIGITAL INTERFACE

Sensors are essentially everywhere. Simplistically, sensors are devices that detect signals, then facilitate the elicitation of a response to the signal. The signals could be physical, chemical, or biological. These could include temperature, pressure, light, touch, weight, fluid levels, magnetic or electric fields, and so on. Our cars, trains, buses, homes, malls, offices, hospitals, and industrial complexes are all and will increasingly be embedded with sensors.

Sensors have little use by themselves. For a sensor to have any role, it has to be part of a larger system. The position of the sensor within the human body or a device can be extrinsic or intrinsic. It may be at the entry point, receiving signals from the outside and informing the device of the external milieu, or a part of the internal circuitry of a larger device. For example, in a car, a sensor monitors functionality and the internal engine state (e.g., tire pressure, oil levels, and brakes). The sensor senses the altered stimuli, acquires the data, then as a component of a larger system, enables feedback.

Like an automobile, the human body can be digitized. Each organ system can be broken down into its multiple functions, with "external sensors" to monitor each one of them. This could provide us with the opportunity for continuous monitoring and proactive interventions to prevent disease. Advances in computing power will enable health care professionals to make minute-by-minute decisions as we follow the varied trajectories of our patients beyond the doctor's office. Sensors will change the way we practice medicine, making care more efficient, objective, quantitative, affordable, and sensible.

We still live in a mostly analog world. Signals from our world need to communicate with the digital world. It is here that sensors constitute the interface between the analog signals (e.g., physical stimuli) and downstream electronic circuits, to which they communicate through generating electrical charges. Sensors are components within any device that uses a digital signal processor. The processor receives the electrical signal and transmits it or generates a response. These microprocessors are an integral part of all computerized appliances, be they cars, planes, thermostats, microwave ovens, or coffee makers. This information is transmitted through streaming electrons. The sensor serves as an interpreter and helps construct a common language between the analog stimulus and the device that it interfaces with. In the world of medicine, sensors now enable the monitoring of vital signs and disease states. Technology has progressed to develop smart sensors that have not only sensing capabilities but also data-processing capabilities to enable a smart response.

SO HOW DOES IT ALL WORK?

Outside the human body, sensors have been described as eyes, ears, and noses derived from silicon chips. The sensor converts stimuli such as heat, light, sound, or motion into electrical signals that are converted into a binary code and sent forward, usually to a computer processor integrated into an electronic system that helps initiate a response or a resulting impulse. From the medical perspective, sensors are sophisticated devices capable of converting physical parameters such as temperature, blood pressure, heart rate, heart sounds, and so on into a signal that can be measured and then transmitted via electrical signals to initiate a response. Collectively, working sensors can routinely send in data of the magnitude of ten gigabytes per second, four hundred times faster than conventional internet speed. Based on the functionality desired, more sensors and increased speed can be added.

These sensors can be complex yet integrated to work together. We know that some cars now have sensory systems that can alert drivers to the onset of drowsiness—for example, through a sensor measuring eyeball movement, head inclination, or grasp on the steering wheel. These sensors are connected with the emergency braking system and aim to enhance safety and take evasive action either through an override option or via advising the driver. Clearly there is no point to having a sensor if there is no effector arm to deploy a response.

In the arena of medicine, the effector arm can be the patient, the health care provider, or a self-contained unit, where the sensor receives the signal that is processed to deliver the desired action. At the patient level, a data point from the sensor such as blood glucose level or a blood pressure measurement alerts the patient to take action. On the other hand, it could be the health care provider who receives the alert and takes the appropriate action. The most highly evolved form of this relationship is the closed-loop system, where the sensor itself initiates the appropriate response—for example, a glucose-sensor-driven insulin release, where the glucose level drives the insulin release from the delivery device. At the other end of the spectrum, there are passive home sensors to monitor for motion and falling. These are installed as environmental sensors and continually feed information either through a smartphone or a wireless modem to a remote-monitoring server that can alert caregivers if there is any change in gait or stability in someone with a propensity to fall.

GOING UPSTREAM IN THE CARE PATHWAY

I have always felt that the need for surgical intervention reflects our inability to tackle a disease through minimally invasive approaches, and/or a lack of understanding at the molecular level that prevents the use of noninvasive pharmacological approaches. We fix things after they are broken or just about to break. The future is dependent upon us continuing to go upstream, so that anything invasive, anything that requires breaking or cutting through skin, becomes archaic. It is here that sensors will provide us with a better understanding and assist upstream disease-modifying measures.

Wearable sensors provide a way to move away from the need to break skin, and provide uninterrupted chemical monitoring using saliva, tears, and sweat, all easily available biological fluids, similar to an oil check with more sophisticated automatic diagnostics. Multiple wearables and implantables may be required in the same patient to monitor different organ systems. This array of sensors will need to work together, so when the check-engine light goes on, we know where to look.

Developing digital sensors that work well is a complex process and comprises the collaborative efforts of a clinician, a sensor engineer, data scientists, and clinical researchers to work toward identifying the unmet need for a clinical condition and then collectively solving it. Sensor development is an iterative process requiring continuous validation and refinement, and may involve not just the biomechanics and electrical circuitry of the sensor but also the feedback loop and algorithm supporting its function.

CAR CARE ANALOGY

Medical costs continue to climb exponentially, and three of every four dollars in the health care budget are now spent on the care of patients with chronic diseases. Concurrent with this are the growing demand for value and a heightened attention to providing patient-centric care. Progressive digitization of the health care industry and electronic health records becoming the norm is forcibly nudging us to think beyond the predictable pattern of clinical care. There is a huge push in health care to shift less-complex care of inpatients to the outpatient arena and the upkeep of our ostensibly clinically straightforward outpatients to their homes. Many of these care aspirations hinge on the increasing pervasiveness of wearables and implanted devices, which provide continuous streaming of physiological data.

Simultaneously, there is an impending need for a culture change in our clinical practice, from the conventional care model that is episodic and transactional to one of continuous care. Even though we see patients at specific time intervals, disease states don't exactly follow the pattern of our clinic visits—patients don't fall ill at three-, six-, or twelve-month intervals. Through these advances in the digital world, being able to deliver the right care at the right time and at the right place to our patients seems closer to becoming a reality.

As stated earlier, the human body can be equated to the automobile, where many sensors are generating, analyzing, and making decisions based on large amounts of digital data. These decisions can be second-to-second, involving the fine-tuning of an engine, or longer term, with periodic maintenance-check lights indicating the need for an elective checkup. Similarly, every organ system can be monitored via sensors, streaming data that are being transmitted on a continual basis. As an electrophysiologist, I have been implanting electrical devices in patients for the last couple of decades. These devices, whether defibrillators or pacemakers, have within them a host of simple sensors that derive their information from heart rate, respiration, heart sounds, physical activity, and impedance measures. (Impedance is a measure of resistance to an electric current within the chest wall and can be significantly abnormal when fluid accumulates within the lungs.) Many of these variables, either individually or combined, can detect and predict life-threatening events. As I will describe in subsequent chapters, these sensors are getting progressively more sophisticated. Just like the check-engine light before a potential breakdown or a call for service, sensors may soon serve to provide a check-organ status light.

WHERE DO WEARABLE DEVICES AND SENSORS FIT INTO THIS EQUATION?

Wearable devices and sensors are part of a complicated landscape that continues to be inundated with new devices and apps. There are already more than half a million health apps and several hundred wearable devices available worldwide. Of these, activity monitors, Fitbits, and smartwatches constitute just a small percentage of devices that can provide on-the-go medical monitoring. Although most apps were initially focused on wellness, there has been an increase in those to monitor disease states. These wearable devices and apps provide us with sensor approaches to help monitor heart rate, blood pressure, temperature, activity, hydration status, sleep stages, stress, and even blood glucose levels. Although these devices have created a wide range of possibilities, they bring with them several challenges, including the reproducibility of the measurements and their integration into the workflow of clinical practice. Also, there are many steps between the sensor activation and the creation of clinically actionable data.

Empowering patients to self-manage their own disease states by using wearable sensor data to detect subtle changes before they become overtly symptomatic is a worthy goal. Nonetheless, much of this will be dependent on better sensors, more accurate and reliable data, and most notably a transformation in the culture of care.

2

DOC-IN-THE-BOX

Anything can change because the smartphone revolution is still in the early stages.
TIM COOK

If I asked you to picture a 103-year-old woman, Beverly likely would not resemble the image that comes to mind. Looking at her lifestyle alone, you'd never know she was my oldest patient. She still drives. She babysits her youngest great-grandchild twice a week. She's tiny, coming in just shy of five feet and hovering around eighty pounds, but what she lacks in physical mass, she compensates for with wit and a perpetual readiness for a good conversation. Beverly has been coming to see me for ten years. While she's the picture of health in many ways, she has been on blood thinners to prevent a recurrence of the stroke she had nearly two decades ago, and she lives in fear of falling and bleeding out because of the medications she takes to prevent clotting.

Over the past ten years, I've grown intimately acquainted not only with Beverly's medical anxieties but with her family. An appointment with Beverly necessarily includes a photo-sharing session. You may be picturing fumbling hands digging through an oversize purse for a stack of printed photos. If so, you'd be entirely off the mark. Instead, Beverly whips out her iPhone, clad in the bright-pink, flower-covered case given to her by Erika, one of her seventeen great-grandchildren. With glee, she confidently navigates the device, rapidly swiping through dozens of pictures while rattling off detailed updates on four generations of family members. This is how it's been since she first came in: Beverly has a smartphone, one regularly updated by the family, that she has fully embraced as her sentinel, as a treasured way to keep connected with her rapidly growing network of offspring.

This is not an isolated example. Half a world away in Delhi, my nearly ninety-year-old mother-in-law, Padma, will not so much as step out of bed in the morning without her smartphone in hand. If she moves room to room throughout the house, so does her phone. It is her lifeline, the means by which she stays connected to her three doting daughters. It is what holds her favorite music and what brings her the latest Bollywood news in real time. And it has become a tool that supplements her traditional health care. During the pandemic, Padma used her smartphone to video call her personal doctor on multiple occasions, which proved invaluable. Perhaps less beneficially, she has also learned how to look up her medications and their side effects online; coincidentally, she then seems to begin experiencing just about all of them. While she's been a smartphone user for years now, it's still hard for me to truly comprehend the ease with which Padma, a lifelong technophobe, can navigate a handheld supercomputer.

On a global scale, the percentage of adults who have a smartphone is rapidly rising as the barriers of age and socioeconomic status shrink. Their increasing accessibility and widespread adoption have resulted in functionalities beyond the wildest dreams of those who remember phones as rudimentary devices that received and enabled audio calls. For many people, smartphones have now replaced cameras, alarm clocks, and calculators. They count our steps, guide us to our destinations, and allow us to bank online. Want to catch up on the news? Check the weather forecast for tomorrow? See the photos from your friend's trip? So many parts of daily life point straight back to the smartphone that can be found clutched in nearly every hand.

Given this rapid trajectory, it shouldn't seem a stretch that the powerful, increasingly ubiquitous device is becoming an integral part of patients' medical care. The widespread social distancing adopted as a result of the COVID-19 pandemic exacerbated a trend already taking shape; like Padma, people around the world relied on video calls to interact with their doctors from a distance. The increase in demand resulted in the video chat function and its availability evolving and being refined at an unprecedented pace.

Yet while this facet alone would have been hard for Beverly or Padma to dream of in their youth, video appointments are only the beginning. Smartphones are now capable of monitoring, predicting, and even preventing disease, thanks to the array of sensors that are built into nearly all models currently available. The uses these sensors can be put to are already vast, even as they're in the dawn of their implementation; they generate, collect, and share data through sophisticated cloud servers, where high-tech algorithms are able to generate personalized care in real time. Smartphones can help people diagnose their ailments, manage their health, and find actionable direction for further care. They are set to become a true doc-in-the-box, radically changing society's approach to illness, whether acute or chronic, mild or severe.

SMARTPHONE SENSORS

Maybe you're exhilarated by this idea. Maybe you're somewhat skeptical. Either way, understanding the staggering medical potential of the smartphone relies on a better understanding of how the built-in sensors work. Their data collection is carried out by three major sensors that independently gauge movement, rotation, and magnetic drift. Separately, each of the three is able to sense and measure various clinical data points that reflect the user's well-being, including heart rate, body contours, energy expenditure, and even sleep patterns. When we look at the data gathered from all three sensors together, we're presented with a comprehensive record of the carrier's vital signs, physical activity, energy consumption, and—very soon, it seems—the function of every organ in the human body.

While it's easy to get excited by the breadth of what is soon to be possible, there are many health applications of the smartphone already in play today at which we can marvel. Take, for example, the photoplethysmography (PPG) capabilities built into nearly every device. PPG can gather crucial data about heart rate and rhythm through contact with the bare skin of a fingertip, ear, or face using the physics of light absorption and reflection. The information around heart rate and heart rate variability gathered through this means has been demonstrated to stack up to commercial ECG monitoring strategies. PPG can also measure the brain/heart connection, blood pressure, and oxygen saturation, as well as facilitate readouts of colorimetric tests on body fluids such as saliva, sweat, and urine.

There are countless ways that organ-specific diagnostic tools can be fashioned around these sensors. Microphones can serve as a spirometer, a breathing instrument used to measure lung function or track voice changes to diagnose heart failure or respiratory distress. Cameras on both the front and back of the smartphone can be used to corroborate heart rate information and measure a user's respiratory rate by examining the chest and abdomen. There are now even contact-free PPG algorithms that can estimate the heart rate and deduce other calculations through examining the user's face. An app called FaceBeat uses the light reflected from the face to assess blood patterns, giving insight into changes in flow or volume. While this technology may sound spectacular, I'd be remiss not to acknowledge that it presents certain challenges. The data in real-life situations may not be collected in as carefully cultivated an environment as it would be in a clinical setting; as such, it's important for users to remember the readings may not be entirely accurate. To illustrate this point, consider the many extrinsic factors that could interfere with the conclusions of FaceBeat: hairstyles covering part of the face, insufficient or irregular lighting, different skin tones, unexpected facial hair, a strange hat—the list goes on.

In addition to the sensors already built into smartphones, there are others that can be worn or implanted to supplement the already high level of data collection possible through the handheld device. Oftentimes, these additional sensors are dedicated to measuring a single variable and therefore tracking and providing more detailed information with the help of a related app on the smartphone. A prime example is the continuous blood glucose sensor that allows a patient to better track and treat their diabetes. Wearable sensors also provide information that a phone stored in the pocket may not be able to consistently provide. For example, wearables such as watches have PPG sensors that are, quite literally, on the pulse and able to deliver real-time information from the outside world to the central command station embedded in the smartphone. The processing ability stored in the small device to which we have all grown so accustomed is staggering.

TRACKING AND TREATING DISEASE

So smartphones can keep detailed records of just about every human function. Great. What, then, do we do with that information? The answer to that question, as you may have come to expect, is expansive, but what it boils down to is this: smartphone sensors provide an opportunity for highly individualized and proactive care, often referred to as *precision medicine*.

Consider the pacing of care provided via conventional practice. Typically, the initial tests, diagnosis, treatment plan, and subsequent adjustments of medication occur over multiple visits spread across weeks, if not months. In contrast, the streaming data available through our smartphones or other wearable sensors dramatically reduces the time it takes to recognize abnormal readings and respond as needed. Before long, we'll be measuring the various steps of treatment in days, then hours, and eventually minutes. Decisions will be expedited through the assistance of health care navigators using AI algorithm-facilitated prescriptive care. Also, much of the care will be automated through informed self-management approaches for patients, and in other situations the implantable device itself may mete out the therapy through a closed-loop system.

While we've established that smartphones are able to gather key insights around a user's health, quantifying risks, detecting issues, and contributing to tailored treatment plans, would you believe me if I told you smartphones can help us predict everything from sudden death to lung disorders to serious mental health problems? Research has shown that smartphones can transmit and process ECG signals on the body's surface, helping to identify life-threatening arrhythmias—irregular beating of the heart—in seemingly healthy patients, creating the opportunity for preventive action to be taken before a serious cardiac event occurs.

If that isn't enough to wow you, let's move on to the lungs. Air pollution is a significant health problem across the globe, contributing to a range of ailments: chronic obstructive lung disease, emphysema, bronchitis, pneumonias, and even lung cancer. The deterioration of lung health is often accompanied by a progressive decline of function, reduced quality of life, and higher death rates. This fluctuation in lung function, paired with certain behavioral patterns, can be detected by a smartphone's sensors. As mentioned earlier, the microphone on a smartphone can be used as a low-cost spirometer. Certain easily downloadable apps can record the audio of a forced exhale and, over time, build out a user's daily breathing pattern and store it on a remote server. The flow rate can then be analyzed and compared to the previously recorded baseline from the patient. Add in oxygen saturation, audio recordings of coughs or exhalation patterns, and AI-based recognition of breathing profiles, and the technology could well catch a flare-up of a lung disorder in its incipient stage.

High-touch technology via smartphones is making it easier to track and treat diseases. There is perhaps no area of medical care that illustrates this point more clearly than that of mental health. It is an unfortunate truth that the social stigma around seeking mental health help has left many who would have deeply benefited from the care to their own devices. Now, however, after generations of quiet struggle, virtual care being made widely accessible through smartphones has helped remove the barrier of shame. From anywhere in the world, a smartphone can be used to discreetly access professional help.

As an extension of this, the use of video-enabled tablets by rurally based US veterans has increased access, with a surge in psychotherapy visits resulting in reduced suicide behavior and emergency room visits.

Notably, the mental health implications don't stop there. Smartphones can also help contribute to the objective assessment of a patient seeking mental health support. Data from the embedded sensors can provide information regarding physical activity, phone usage, and sleep patterns, both actively and passively collecting data that sheds light on the user's mental state. Smartphones can even enable the digital phenotyping or characterization of behavioral patterns in depressive behavior and detect changes from the norm. Sudden aberrations in the daily information can reflect fluctuations in anxiety levels and have proven specifically useful for diagnosing and monitoring depression, bipolar disorder, autism, and schizophrenia. Systems such as CrossCheck can use data from a phone's sensors, call history, and phone usage to identify patterns that can predict changes in mental health in schizophrenia patients. Researchers recently launched an app called Autism & Beyond, which runs facial expressions captured by smartphone cameras through an algorithm to help the user with emotional categorization. External sensors that function largely on their own have proven ideal for younger autistic children, such as a smartwatch that changes color to indicate the child is upset based on changes it detects in heart or respiratory rate.

I was again reminded of the value of data derived from smartphones when, in a recent discussion, a psychiatrist colleague of mine said, "The phone doesn't lie." While it may not give you all the information you wish it did, what it does provide is an unfiltered representation of the user's physical and mental state of being. How to best interpret the raw data is still being determined; currently, the most widely accepted practice is to compare the data from unwell patients to their own data from periods of so-called normalcy. This type of characterization, based on data aggregated from the different sensors in the smartphone, seems to be more precise than self-reporting.

WEARABLES: NOVEL OR VITAL?

When I think of wearable sensors, I think of Louise. Louise was a portly, sixty-three-year-old medical assistant of Irish origin who loved her job, loved her grandchildren, and loved her Fitbit—an activity-tracking device that, of its many functionalities, is best known for counting steps. As a medical assistant, Louise was responsible for ushering patients back and forth from the waiting room to the clinic offices, where she'd take their vital signs, record an ECG, and make sure that the room was turned over and ready for the next patient when the appointment was finished. With more than three hundred patients coming through daily, Louise was a frenzy of activity, and she was absolutely obsessed with getting her step count up. Some days, we'd make it a competition to see who could walk more. She beat me every single time, usually winning by a margin of four thousand steps or more. She did the hard work while I was busy pontificating with patients. I knew it wasn't just a game for Louise; she was committed to staying healthy. Sadly, her robust step count proved no match to the cancer that claimed her life.

I want to be clear: high step counts are good, and measuring physical activity is important, but we need to be wary of relying on a single variable to assess our well-being when dozens of factors work together to indicate good or bad health. Taken at face value, a step count divulges very little beyond determining whether a user is sedentary or active. For external wearables to be put to their most comprehensive and accurate use, users must take a step back and consider the bigger picture.

Steps can be examined in several ways. From the spatial perspective alone, we can derive in-depth information that is routinely overlooked. Temporal variables such as stride length, step width, speed, and acceleration can be used to monitor average activity, joint health, and fall risk. Using time as a metric, we can weigh up stop time, stance time, stride time, and cadence to monitor for specific disease states. For example, Parkinson's disease, a neuromuscular disorder, can be diagnosed and then stratified for its severity by very typical gait changes. The gait in Parkinson's disease transforms over a period to one that is associated with small, shuffling steps and slowing movement. Beyond this, a patient's activity level can also be a determinant of frailty or illness and flag the existence of other neuropathic conditions and muscular dystrophies that affect gait and steadiness. It's important to note, however, that the absence of activity can tell as much as, if not more than, the activity that is recorded. Significant drops in—or even total cessation of—activity are often evidenced in patients with depression, while a marked increase in activity may be a sign a patient is in a manic phase of their mental disorder.

Wearable sensors have been linked to the identification of other common ailments, such as hypertension and diabetes. When doctors catch and address these conditions early on, patients may avoid devastating future consequences altogether. Already, clinicians have begun to adopt wearables to facilitate and refine many of the fundamentals of health care: Heart rate can be accurately measured via wearables on the finger, wrist, arm, ear, neck, or chest. Blood oxygen saturation—a metric used to monitor patients at home to ascertain when and whether they need to be brought into the hospital—can be recorded noninvasively from the fingertip or the earlobe. Patients' respiration rate, blood pressure, and temperature can each be determined with ease, regularity, and accuracy via wearables, providing timely and constantly updated insight into how sick they may actually be. The progress in this space is rapid, and an expanding array of sensors means cancer, lung disease, neurological disorders, and more are inching their way onto the list of diseases able to be detected through such monitoring.

We are still in the early days of wearable technology. While it has found inroads into certain consumer groups, adoption is largely concentrated among fitness enthusiasts and wellness groups. For those pushing the technology forward, the hope is that wearables will become more widespread among consumers and that the information, combined with the data collected by smartphones, will be integrated with data from implantables and collectively build out an electronic medical record. The hope is that as this technology continues to be adopted, it will become a formalized part of the health care pathway, not only providing doctors with real-time patient information but feeding AI-algorithms free-flowing, continuous data—radically transforming the way we practice medicine.

MAKING A FASHION STATEMENT

It's hardly hyperbole to say there is no limit to the ways in which wearable sensors can be worn, especially given the pace of innovation in the space. Every day new products hit the market that can be affixed to heads, necks, torsos, ears, arms, and legs. They can be applied either directly to the skin or attached to clothes but are largely designed to blend into a normal wardrobe, taking the shape of glasses, hats, earrings, earbuds, necklaces, or headbands.

Chic earrings can monitor temperature, oxygen saturation, and physical activity. Microchips in earbuds can measure the heart and respiratory rate from filling capillaries, blood pressure, and core body temperature from within the ear canal. Mouthguards for sports or sleep issues can use sensors to extract enzymatic data from saliva. Smart hats can monitor most physiological parameters and even measure brain activity, helping to deliver actionable insights that improve the user's life. Take, for example, the ability to monitor brain activity occurring during unintended sleep that affects work performance and causes accidents.

Smart glasses, operated by voice command and able to measure heart rate, physical activity, and temperature, are now masquerading as trendy tortoiseshell frames. They may contain a host of sensors, such as accelerometers and microphones, and are even able to help with the readouts of colorimetric tests from body fluids such as saliva, sweat, blood, or urine, but the technology is compact and discreet. If glasses don't fit somebody's style, there's no need to fret. Smart contact lenses, fitted snugly to the eye, can still contain temperature and pressure sensors, helping to monitor eye diseases such as glaucoma. Lenses that can monitor glucose levels in tears are currently being tested, a development that would prove incredibly helpful in regulating diabetes.

The wearable market is focusing much of its energy on similarly noninvasive technology. The future, it seems, is smart fabrics. As embedding textiles with tiny electronic sensors continues to catch on, everything you wear could contribute to a real-time reading of the state of your personal engine. Because stretchable electronics are able to conform to the body and can bend, twist, and expand along with natural motions, they maintain skin-to-skin contact and transmit high-fidelity signals that pick up heart rate, respiratory rate, and ECG signals with great accuracy. Smart fabrics can measure variation in force, pressure, humidity, and body temperature, while also tracking muscle activity and posture. Again, the usage extends far beyond measuring performance. Radiofrequency sensors can help detect the presence of fluid in the lungs, for example, which is valuable for patients at risk of heart failure or dealing with lung disease. Assuming user adoption, organ-specific information will be available for all states of being while working, eating, exercising, and sleeping via smart shirts, shoes, bras, vests, swimsuits . . . even socks, the humblest piece of a wardrobe. Smart socks can provide a 3D representation of pressure distribution during walking, generating feedback to inform orthopedic problems—especially useful in patients who have pressure sores or a diabetic foot syndrome. Sensors in the insoles communicate each heel strike to the watch, aiding athletes to understand their stride and prevent stress injuries and fractures. Many diabetics experience a narrowing of their blood vessels, reducing blood supply to the limbs and causing ulceration of the foot. They are also prone to developing nerve disease, which can result in the loss of sensation in the lower extremities. The guidance made possible by smart socks helps patients and their caregivers individualize care to prevent these outcomes and minimize further injuries.

Smart fabrics are also ideally suited to fully utilize the gold mine of information presented by body fluids, a source of knowledge that is often unplumbed, as handling bodily fluids such as sweat, tears, and urine can prove challenging—especially during a pandemic. Such fluids can, however, be key in diagnosing and informing the treatment of several widespread, chronic diseases that afflict millions of patients. Through sweat alone, one can diagnose diseases such as diabetes, electrolyte abnormalities, and even autonomic nervous system diseases in certain cases.

One such detectable ailment is cystic fibrosis, a progressive genetic disease that affects the cells that produce mucus, sweat, and digestive juices, resulting in the buildup of mucus in the lungs to the point of obstruction, infections, and premature death. With smart fabrics, it is easy to measure the pH of a user's sweat. While the pH of a healthy person will come in between 4.5 to 6.5, that of a patient with cystic fibrosis can be as high as 9.0. New stretchable pH sensors can take this reading and directly communicate it to the user's smartphone, allowing for real-time medication adjustments as needed. What the pH of a user's sweat can tell us doesn't stop there. It can inform hydration and physiological status in athletes, helping to bolster performance. It can be useful for monitoring chronic wounds, as pH levels help to determine a user's response to specific treatments. It plays a part in treating and monitoring skin disorders such as dermatitis and fungal infections.

All this is possible, and we have covered just one aspect of one body fluid, and not exhaustively at that. I haven't even mentioned the tattoo sensors that can be drawn out on paper and stuck to the skin, providing highly accurate monitoring of a range of vital biophysical and biochemical signals. Or the wireless, flexible, bio-integrated skin sensors that are compatible with low-cost mobile phones. Or sensor-studded patches and badges that can monitor vital signs and track heart failure, pneumonia, lung disease, and urinary tract and other infections while patients are at home. These cheap, highly customizable products are all poised to contribute to the deployment of wearables at scale in lower- and middle-income countries where resources and personnel are limited.

Cost, customizability, coolness, and how well they fit into the larger picture of a patient's care will determine which of these technologies become most prevalent. Ultimately, the products that are comfortable, washable, reusable, rechargeable, and—most importantly—scalable will win out.

THE WEARABLE WORLD OF TOMORROW

The world of wearables is new and experimental, with nearly every vendor in the space adopting a different technique and following a unique strategy with their sensors, complicating how they are able to contribute usable data into one cohesive, digestible patient file. Assimilating the many approaches into a streamlined electronic medical record system will take time.

Ongoing discussion also wages around when, if ever, wearable sensors should be classified as medical devices. The boundary between a fitness or wellness app and a medical app is becoming increasingly unclear and is further muddied by the fact that self-monitoring is not yet considered part of the conventional care pathway. Concern lingers over the substantial amount of user awareness and intentionality necessary for sensors to be truly effective and beneficial. Inconsistent use and the appearance of unexpected environmental variables can easily foster reliance upon inaccurate measurements, ultimately leading to user harm. This could be in the form of unnecessary changes to medications or modifying one's activity based on erroneous data.

How can we facilitate individualized calibration of devices for different body types, with valid clinical tools that can serve as the gold standard? How do we quantify and factor in misreadings that are sure to be triggered by external influences? How do we minimize unpredictable variables? For the data coming from the wearable sensors to be of value, we must be able to answer these questions about the trustworthiness of the signal and the reproducibility of the methodology.

There are larger, overarching concerns that stand separate from the science of the sensors themselves. Sure, they need to be tested, but they also need to be affordable. Ideally, they'll be integrated across all processing systems. Then, even when the science is sound, the wearable must be comfortable enough and the app user-friendly enough to draw people in. On top of the need for marketing, pushing adoption, and retaining users loom big questions around privacy and security; there are undoubtedly many open questions to be answered.

Addressing those barriers one by one may seem daunting. It may even seem impossible. But imagine, if you will, that we were able to step back to 1938. That we were able to sit down with a twenty-year-old Beverly and say, "In your lifetime, you will own not one, but many supercomputers. Devices so small you can hold one in your hand, until you toss it away for a newer, faster, better model. This computer will know everything about you, inside and out. It will interact with other technology elsewhere on your person, in your home, and around the world. It will become a partner to your in-person doctor and the command station from which you run your life."

She'd laugh you out of the room.

So then, what grounds are there to doubt that our human intelligence, bolstered by a supercomputer in every palm, will usher in a new era of personalized medicine?

3

THE FAILING HEART, THE DYING PATIENT, AND IMPLANTABLE SENSORS

A mining engineer does not assay a mountain of ore by testing one rock.

NORMAN JEFFERIS HOLTER

Laura found herself gasping for breath after minimal movement. Her breathing was getting progressively worse. Even getting off the bed was challenging. To be able to breathe better, she had to prop herself up in bed with a couple of pillows. This helped reduce the pressure on her lungs and allowed her to take deeper breaths. Leaning forward helped her lungs expand a tad better, and she spent most of the afternoon sitting up in her recliner. She feared she might need to do that all night.

Laura was forty-two years old with a history of heart failure from a weakened heart muscle due to a viral infection she contracted six years ago. Doctors had never clearly explained to her why this transpired or why her heart function had continued to decline over the past few years, though they did tell her that people with weak hearts like hers can have a very rapid decline and most often don't survive. They called it giant cell myocarditis, a fulminant inflammation of the heart muscle that acutely causes the heart to fail. Four years ago, she was implanted with a defibrillator, a small metallic device inserted into her chest wall to protect her from any life-threatening heart-rhythm disturbance. A potentially fatal heart rhythm could be automatically detected by the device, which would then electrically jolt her heart back into its normal state. She was told that if things did not turn around, she would die from either a deadly arrhythmia or progressive heart failure, or maybe both at the same time.

She felt lucky to be alive; however, right now she didn't feel all that lucky. Her breathing was getting more labored, despite her taking her medicines and doing all the things Dr. Parks had asked her to do. She felt responsible for her current situation and almost like a hypochondriac. She couldn't figure out why she felt so ill, as she had seen the nurse practitioner just last week in person. She had been examined carefully, and her medication doses had been adjusted. Laura convinced herself that she would be fine. She could still walk to the bathroom and to her kitchen, all on the same level, and could take care of herself. She did not want to bother her neighbors and clearly felt that she was not sick enough to call 911. So Laura did what she thought was best. She rested and hoped it would all go away, just like a bad cold.

Fast-forward twenty-four hours, and Laura was now profoundly short of breath. Her breathing was shallow, making a rattling sound, and her speech was fragmented. She was unable to speak in full sentences, as she had to catch her breath between words. When Laura called 911, it did not take more than a few seconds for the EMTs to realize that she was in florid heart failure. When they arrived, she was coughing up red, frothy sputum, and her lungs were full of fluid. She gasped for breath as the EMTs fitted her with a face mask providing 100 percent oxygen and an intravenous line to push diuretics. The intention was to help take some fluid off, quickly, to ease her breathing while they made their way to the hospital. Laura was now sweating profusely, and her breathing continued to get shallower and more rapid. Her oxygen saturation had dropped to 78 percent.

She does not remember passing out before she reached the hospital or the physicians and nursing team gathering around her as she arrived in the ER, where like a well-oiled machine, they passed an endotracheal tube down her throat and connected that to a ventilator. Her oxygen levels quickly rose back to the nineties as she lay on the hospital bed in the ER, sedated on a ventilator with multiple plastic tubes running from her arms to IV poles flanking her on either side. She had been just a few minutes away from what could have been a fatal event. So many things went wrong here. The downhill spiral could have been caught early on and mitigated. Although this clinical scenario is quite avoidable, the same situation repeats itself with thousands of patients daily.

THE PROBLEM

Heart failure poses a huge clinical and economic burden. It affects more than 6.5 million Americans and is the leading cause of hospitalization among people over the age of sixty-five. Importantly, a weak heart muscle is now a primary public health concern, and hospitalization expenses for the management of thousands of acute decompensations in patients every day imposes a substantial financial burden on the health care system. When patients get admitted, they often need several days of monitoring in the critical care unit or a sophisticated unit with arrhythmia monitoring. The use of resources is quite intense. There are more than half a million new cases of heart failure each year, with cumulatively more than seven million "hospitalizations days" per year.

This disease drains the national treasury by more than $40 billion on an annual basis, and the projected expenditure by the health care system overall is $70 billion by 2030. With each subsequent admission, the patient never really bounces back to their prior clinical state; they are always a little sicker than before. The clinical trajectory becomes set on a downhill course. Of note, the vast majority of these patients admitted with decompensated heart failure are known to the medical system and to medical providers, thereby creating an opportunity for upstream strategies that may be capable of detecting the failing heart early in its course and implementing therapies to stabilize the patient and avert hospitalization. When such proactive care is delivered, it prevents the progression of heart failure, improves long-term clinical outcomes, and lowers death rates.

The concept of outpatient remote monitoring for early detection and treatment of worsening heart function is not new; however, the lack of clarity on which parameters to monitor and how they should be used to prevent hospitalization has continued to plague the health care system for the last decade or more. Usually, as in Laura's case, when the patient develops clinical symptoms and overt signs of heart failure, it is often too late. The damage may already have been done, and recovery may never be complete.

It is quite strange that despite all the advances in medical and device therapy over the last thirty years, treating and stabilizing the failing heart remains problematic. This is despite us knowing that heart failure is probably the most common final pathway for most people who have heart disease. At any given time, at least 10 percent or more of the patients admitted to a tertiary hospital setting carry the diagnosis of heart failure. Notably, if one is lucky enough to get old and not get cancer, then probably one will see some form of heart failure along the course of one's life. Heart failure can come in many forms; it may range from a mild increase in shortness of breath to an extreme—as in Laura's situation, with florid symptoms requiring intubation and mechanical ventilatory support. It's not that the medical community is ignoring this; it's just that they have not been able to construct a well-oiled, widely accepted disease management platform for this group of patients as of yet. The advent of virtual care and possibility of sensor-aided objectivity to the clinical evaluation seem to offer hope.

SENSOR SOLUTIONS

A big challenge in managing the failing heart is that the classic clinical signs and symptoms to make the diagnosis are not always easily elicitable. Even though the clinical evaluation has a well-regimented protocol that involves measuring the heart rate, respiratory rate, and blood pressure, examining the legs for swelling due to fluid retention, looking at the neck veins to assess the jugular venous distension, or listening to the chest for murmurs and the intensity of the heart sounds, there is considerable subjectivity in this assessment. The routine physical examination, as good as it is, has many limitations.

Other objective measures include direct visualization of the contractile function of the heart via an echocardiogram or a blood test to measure a biomarker such as B-type natriuretic peptide (BNP), which can provide alternative objective measures of the heart function. However, many clinical trials and studies in large patient populations have shown us time and again that a blood test is only a representation of the risk or the clinical state at the time it was measured. Similarly, the echocardiogram is a measurement of the heart function at a snapshot in time. It does not provide a continuous mode of risk stratification that can guide treatment of these vulnerable patients along their unpredictable clinical course.

SO WHERE DO WE GO FROM HERE?

Would it not be phenomenal if we had an implanted sensor within the heart or the body that could help us quickly figure out whether a patient was headed in the wrong direction? Is it crazy to suppose that sensors within the body could help us predict a heart failure episode a month before it actually occurs? Is it out of context to envisage that we should be able to proactively prevent a hospital admission for worsening heart function?

Believe it or not, some of this technology is already here. Most patients with heart failure and low heart function are vulnerable to malignant and often fatal heart-rhythm disturbances. These patients are frequently implanted with pacemakers and defibrillator devices. Laura had such a defibrillator that I had surgically placed in her chest wall under the skin and connected to her heart via insulated electrical wires, which could electrically pace her heart as required and jolt it out of a life-threatening rhythm if needed.

It is not lost on the clinical community that if you implant something in the heart, then it should be able to provide us with information to continuously monitor the patient. And that is exactly what most implanted pacemakers and defibrillators allow us to do. These devices have sensors embedded within them that can measure heart rate, physical activity, respiratory rate, and the buildup of fluid in the lungs. The beat-to-beat variance in the heart rate, known as heart rate variability, is a surrogate for the autonomic tone that is reflective of the brain-heart connection. Heart rate variability is a well-recognized sensor-derived measure of health and predictor of disease. Beyond these, a multitude of high-tech sensors in these implantable devices can measure the intensity of the heart sounds, serving as a stand-in measure for cardiac contractility, and in other cases directly measure the pulmonary artery pressure or left atrial pressure within the heart. As you can imagine, these measures provide more objective information than a simple superficial clinical exam.

The most common causes of heart failure patients having setbacks include the inability to adhere to their medications, lack of understanding of their disease, and shortage of access to care and follow-up visits. Interestingly, administrators have had a single-minded focus on hiring personnel and setting up transition clinics at hospitals, allowing patients to be seen within two weeks of being discharged from the hospital to make sure they don't slip through the cracks and bounce back to the emergency room for recurrent heart failure; however, there is little energy or attention paid to setting up remote-monitoring approaches. Remote monitoring allows for the wireless transmission of these sensor-derived measurements from within the devices directly to the doctor's office. Continuous or even intermittent monitoring of alerts for each of these parameters, coupled with a virtual visit, can obviate the need for a frail, decompensated, usually elderly patient to travel long distances for a short in-person visit. It is not inconceivable that in certain situations, the patients may clinically deteriorate from the stress of the travel, finding parking, and making their way through the labyrinth of a big hospital. Some of Laura's hesitancy was furthered by the intimidation of the entire rigmarole of getting to the hospital and then working her way through the maze of corridors and walkways to get to her doctor's office. Beyond this, the fear of being admitted to the hospital encouraged her procrastination. So she stayed at home, hoping for the best.

REMOTE MONITORING

Some patients with heart failure who have implanted devices can be proactively monitored from a distance. Clinicians and some remote-monitoring centers have the ability to follow data transmitted from sensors within the device on demand. Laura's precipitous clinical decline could have been averted if her sensors were being actively remotely monitored. The increase in her heart rate and respiratory rate, the decline in her physical activity, and the changing intensity of her heart sounds, along with buildup of fluid in her lungs as measured by the sensors within her implanted defibrillator device, could all have been detected several days to weeks before she presented in a critical state. Her medications could have been proactively adjusted a few days prior, and none of this would have happened.

Most doctors, heart failure experts, and institutions are working their hardest to keep the patient healthy and avoid heart failure admissions. An added incentive is trying to stave off federal penalties to hospitals due to readmissions. These institutions are coming up with homegrown risk-scoring strategies based on clinical parameters such as race, age, gender, and comorbidities. Population-based methods using these risk scores rarely work well at the individual level. Every one of us is vastly different from another when one begins to examine the impact of genomic, ethnic, social, environmental, cultural, psychological, and medical influences on our internal milieu and how we manifest with disease. How one responds to external stressors, infections, and illness is very different. Having a continuous measure of a range of clinical variables will provide the opportunity to use the patient as their own control. This is the "N of one" approach, where the patient is compared not to some derived standardized value for the general population but instead to their own self during periods of health. This is the only way forward.

Any deviation from the norm of one or more clinical variables such as heart rate, temperature, respiratory rate, blood pressure, or oxygen saturations will allow early recognition of a changing clinical state, enabling prompt intervention. Implantable devices can provide this information separately for each variable or even as a collective integrated measure of several variables providing an alert to the health care provider. Recent wearable strategies such as the Amazon Halo and the Apple Watch also allow for many of these measures to be tracked. The wearable data does not yet have the same fidelity and continuity as an implantable device but can potentially be a useful adjunct to a clinical evaluation over a virtual channel. This is where medicine is headed.

In recent years there has been a fourfold increase in hospital discharges of heart failure admissions. More importantly, 50 percent of these patients get readmitted, and when they leave the hospital, they leave sicker and more vulnerable for another admission. Each admission chips away at their survival curve. There is evidence to suggest that most of these admissions, at least half, are preventable. Laura is a part of this statistic.

It is self-evident that the use of sensors in her care could have enabled decisions that would have contained the downward spiral. Timely intervention with medication adjustments made remotely could have prevented her from getting intubated and being placed on a ventilator. Laura already had an implanted device with sensors that could have forewarned the clinicians or the patient that an intervention was needed to avert the disaster that resulted. Now, here she was on a ventilator in the hospital; if her diuretic dose had been adjusted a few days earlier, this angst could have been avoided.

ARE INTEGRATING IMPLANTABLE SENSORS THE SOLUTION?

As a cardiac electrophysiologist, I have been dealing with implantable sensors for more than two decades. My interest was piqued at a research meeting at MIT approximately eighteen years ago. The proposal under discussion was implanting loop recorders or sensors in our soldiers, just under the skin, so that they could be easily tracked in enemy territory. The sensors would provide information about heart rate and other vital statistics that could help better define the physical state of the soldier. This would be useful not only to locate them but also to determine whether captured soldiers needed a rescue mission. If sensors could detect the health of our soldiers thousands of miles away in distant lands, why couldn't we use them to look after patients within our immediate geography? The implantable sensor provides the opportunity of monitoring a variety of clinical parameters over a wide spectrum of disease states.

But then, why would anyone want something inserted under their skin if the same information could be obtained using a wearable device or sensor? One of the biggest issues with wearable sensors is adherence. Patients tend to overuse the devices in the beginning and then lose interest. Some of this comes from forgetting or just a lack of enthusiasm toward collecting information that may not be immediately relevant. Some sensors need to be actively in contact with the body and others don't. There are those that can collect information passively from a distance. Sensors fitted into the surroundings can pick up information about gait stability, steps, motion, and so on. There are sensors that can detect cardiac issues and disease states from facial images using AI-based approaches. Just a change in skin tone and patterns of blood flow to the face can be passively picked up by your computer or mobile phone to assist with diagnosis. No wearables needed. These approaches, active or passive, implantable or wearable, are not mutually exclusive; they may all serve to complement each other. So how do we wrap our arms around this?

Implantable devices are embedded with sensors that can detect change in a discrete measurable parameter and signal an effector arm to initiate a response. The effector arm could be an alert to the physician or to the patient to intervene based on the data acquired from the sensor. For example, a change in blood-sugar level detected by a glucose-monitoring sensor alerts the physician or the patient to automatically adjust the dose of insulin. As explained in Part III: Artificial Intelligence, some implantable devices can process the signal and themselves initiate a response, such as releasing a medication from a depot, or providing alternative therapy.

Of a variety of standalone sensors, one can be directly implanted in the pulmonary artery. This provides early evidence of left heart failure, where the pressure in the pulmonary artery begins to rise before the buildup of fluid in the lungs. But again, this picks up signals only after the heart has begun to fail. Are there sensor measures that are more sensitive and upstream that can pick up heart failure really early, based on only mild changes in heart function? A few years ago, I helped lead a study that involved the direct placement of a pressure sensor into the left atrium to measure subtle changes in left atrial pressure. These pressure changes are a very early sign of a decline in cardiac function. At that time, this was a complex procedure that involved us getting access to the venous circulation in the body from the right upper shoulder and the right groin area. Additionally, we used a needle inside the heart, guided by echocardiography, to make a hole between the left and right atrium to thread the sensor clip into the left atrium, where it unfolded and could be tugged against the interatrial septal wall. This served to directly measure the left atrium pressure. It turned out to be a complex procedure resulting in cardiac perforations that caused the study to be halted prematurely for safety reasons. Nevertheless, in the hundreds of patients who had the implant safely, it turned out to be a good predictor of heart failure and enabled more proactive individualized monitoring and early intervention. We were able to cut the rate of hospital readmissions by 30 percent. The system allowed for continuous wireless monitoring of left atrial pressure. The sensor was coupled via a subcutaneous antenna to a handheld patient adviser module (like a cell phone), which contained a range of patient alerts with reminders to take medications or obtain additional left atrial pressure recordings. Additionally, the patient adviser module was able to generate a customized patient prescription including medication dosage, activity level, sodium and fluid intake, and physician contact. The prescription was part of a physician-directed patient self-management program. It was technology a few years ahead of its time.

THE SAGA OF THE FALSE-POSITIVE SIGNAL

Conventional implanted pacemaker or defibrillator devices have simple sensors that can provide information on heart rate, respiratory rate, intensity of heart sounds, physical activity, and transthoracic impedance. The latter is a measure of electrical resistance across the chest wall that can detect fluid accumulation within the lungs, which correlates well with worsening heart failure. Because of its simplicity of use, measuring transthoracic impedance was considered an early breakthrough in monitoring heart failure. There were two problems with this. First, it was downstream to changes in left atrial or pulmonary pressure, and second, it was susceptible to error in certain situations. This becomes especially important as false sensor alarms can increase patient anxiety and health care utilization. This is exactly what happened.

In the recent past, a clinical trial called Diagnostic Outcome Trial in Heart Failure (DOT-HF) was implemented to see whether patient engagement with a sensor approach could help alert patients proactively and prevent a hospital visit. Per the protocol of the clinical study, a predefined change in the extent of the accumulation of fluid in the lung measured via the transthoracic impedance sensor was set to alert the patient with a beep, so the patient could then call the doctor's office and seek advice to prevent a heart failure exacerbation. The results of this trial were quite counterintuitive.

The number of outpatient visits and inpatient admissions increased significantly in the group of patients who were alerted by their device. Why did this happen? The explanation is actually quite simple: the alert was very sensitive but not specific, and as a result, patients were often inappropriately alerted by a beep from their device. Consequently, many patients presumed that they must be in heart failure, even though they had no symptoms and felt quite well. When asked, the patients stated that, to them, "the beep" reflected impending doom. This accentuated their anxiety, and the phone call to their doctors or the ER resulted in unnecessary hospitalization.

Seemingly, the lack of familiarity with this sensor alert among the patients' other caregivers further resulted in this overuse of health care resources. Many of the clinicians functioning as the first responder to the alert had not been educated enough about the false-positive rates and, erring on the side of safety, chose to admit the patients to the hospital. In addition, many of the physicians involved in this arc of care who had received the appropriate education ended up second-guessing themselves. They were not sure whether the sensor knew something more than they did, and worried that they might send a patient home who could come back even sicker. It became a case of defensive medicine. Rather than patients being better managed remotely, they ended up using more hospital resources, contrary to the motive of the clinical study. This embarrassing initial experience highlighted that there are pivotal issues beyond just ensuring patient safety during sensor implantation. The true success of a sensor-based approach is dependent on a carefully crafted care pathway and well-informed clinicians looking after the patient.

THE NEED FOR INTEGRATING SENSORS

After the DOT-HF study, most investigators in the world of sensors quickly realized that the only way to combat the false-positive alerts from a single sensor would be to use more than one sensor (measuring different but related variables) showing a collective trend in the same direction. An integrated multisensor strategy could serve to reduce the false-positive alerts and increase the faith of responding clinicians in the directionality of the alert. I had the privilege of being involved as an adviser in the validation and construction of such a multisensor approach that would be integrated into an implantable device to help identify heart failure flare-ups and prevent admissions. The thought here was, if one used a blended (integrated) sensor strategy, maybe we could get it right. Traditionally, when one examines a patient with heart failure, besides their symptoms, they also demonstrate a battery of clinical signs during a physical examination that helps confirm the diagnosis. These include a faster heart rate, a raised jugular venous pressure caused by the circulation backing up as a result of poor forward flow, and change in the intensity of their heart sounds. Along with this, these patients are short of breath because of the accumulation of fluid in their lungs, so their respiratory rate is higher than normal, and physical activity is less as a result of their symptoms. Now if you put all this together, it becomes quite self-evident that if you can have a battery of sensors in a single device to measure these clinical changes within a patient, then maybe you can predict and prevent heart failure in these patients. That is exactly what transpired.

A proprietary algorithm incorporating sensors to measure the intensity of the heart sounds, respiratory rate, physical activity, heart rate trends, and transthoracic impedance was developed and integrated into a "collective index." If that index rose above a certain threshold, it predicted a high risk for hospital admission. The rate of false positives was now significantly lower, and the prediction of a heart failure event was almost spot-on. It is important to note that most patients who develop symptoms from heart failure do so over time. It is rarely an acute event (although that can also happen), oftentimes incipient and simmering over a few days to weeks till it bubbles over into a florid event that results in a hospitalization that often becomes an emergency, as in Laura's case.

DETECTING THE DECLINE AND PREVENTING HOSPITALIZATIONS

Patients like Laura who require admission usually are very sick by the time they come to the attention of the clinician and need to go straight to the intensive care unit. Here they are often given intravenous diuretics to remove the retained fluid and medications to help the pumping function of a failing heart, with further optimization of their home medicines. There is often an accompanying visit to the catheterization laboratory, where they get catheters threaded into their hearts to measure the intracardiac pressures and examine the overall circulatory state. This results in a usually weeklong hospitalization with many blood draws and sometimes other forms of acute, invasive therapies to salvage the deteriorating situation.

But what if all this could be prevented? What if we could detect the gradual decline many weeks before the seminal hospitalization event? Well, that is actually possible. This integrated index can help predict a heart failure event one month before it occurs. Not only that, but it also has the ability to identify windows of time during which the patient is at a tenfold increased risk for worsening heart failure events. There are some blood tests of biomarkers that are helpful in risk-stratifying patients for heart failure events. One of these, the N-terminal B-type natriuretic peptide (NT-pro-BNP), is a hormone released from the atrium musculature due to the rising pressure within the heart and is currently the benchmark. Some of our research work showed that using this integrated sensor index along with NT-pro-BNP identified time periods with a fiftyfold increased risk of heart failure events. This is quite an advance in the science of prediction!

Alternatively, a noninvasive or wearable way of constructing an integrated signaling strategy could also provide us with a measure of the "true" clinical state. Automatic daily evaluation from these sensors via a smartwatch could help demonstrate a trend that could be compared with the patient's own baseline, providing a more elegant, individualized risk-stratification approach. Many clinical studies are starting to examine the logistics and added value of this approach over the conventional follow-up visit. There are some things in medicine that just make clear sense, and this is one of those situations. Not everything needs an elaborate, prohibitively expensive randomized clinical trial of thousands of patients. Rather than waiting, I have personally already started using smartwatch data to manage some of my patients with heart failure and other clinical conditions. It is very individualized at this stage.

On several occasions, this has allowed timely interventions to mitigate a clinical decline or avoid an ER visit. An example that immediately comes to mind is Michael, a forty-eight-year-old CEO of a software start-up in Cambridge, Massachusetts. Michael was diagnosed with a genetic disorder known as Lamin A/C cardiomyopathy about ten years ago. This put Michael at increased risk for heart failure and sudden death. What impressed me most about Michael was how he took all this in stride and never wavered in his personal ambition, lifestyle, or even exercise routine. He continues to run his company of over forty-five employees and spend as much time as he can with his two teenage daughters. He usually works out daily for an hour, of which forty minutes are on his Peloton bike. He recently noticed that even though his effort tolerance was the same as before, he had to catch his breath a little more. He did not make much of this, and it was difficult for me to objectively quantify. Most insightful, however, was his perception of his resting heart rate; this was usually between fifty and fifty-five beats per minute but was now consistently between seventy and seventy-five. This was new. Although this could still be considered a normal heart rate, it was different from his baseline of the past several years. It was unlikely to be related to aging since growing old is usually accompanied by a slowing of the heart rate. A persistent increase in the resting heart rate was a subtle indication that Michael's heart failure may be progressing. An echocardiogram confirmed our suspicion. His heart function had clearly declined, and we needed to bolster his medical regimen. A simple yet objective categorization of his baseline heart rate from a smartwatch was all we needed to tweak his treatment plan to prevent any further decline. Michael continues to do well and inspire me (and others around him) each time I get to meet him during a clinic visit.

CLOSING THE LOOP

To date, most sensor strategies have transmitted clinical information to the health care provider, who is then responsible for "closing the loop" by implementing an appropriate therapeutic intervention. This strategy has several limitations, including the potential for time lags between the sensed event and the implementation of the appropriate intervention. Additionally, a health care provider is still required to interpret the data and make appropriate clinical decisions, which may require substantial resources. Alternatively, information from implanted sensors may be relayed directly to the patient, who then serves as the primary effector; however, patient-driven strategies suffer from variability in patient capability, literacy, and compliance. Additionally, this poses the need for simple decision-making algorithms enabling self-management approaches. Patients will need to interpret the information from the sensor and take an extra pill or modify their lifestyle. This will still need to be prescriptive and individualized. Perhaps the greatest potential of implantable devices with sensors lies in the ability to couple both sensor and effector functions within the device.

This strategy would allow for a truly closed-loop system, which would eliminate dependence on human factors. Additionally, the sensor-effector unit could work in an iterative fashion, with the sensor able to measure the response to a particular intervention and then make further changes based on the dynamic nature of the disease. For instance, there is great interest in the development of microelectromechanical systems (MEMS) capable of controlled drug delivery via an implantable device. It's conceivable that the timely and potentially localized delivery of various pharmacologic agents (e.g., diuretics, steroids, chemotherapeutic agents, or antidiabetic drugs) could serve as a useful individualized treatment modality with a feedback loop. Implantable sensors will become part of routine clinical care and, when coupled with remote monitoring, will allow the practice of a more personalized form of medicine. Some of this is already happening in its early stages with the administration of agents to control blood pressure, glucose level, and pulmonary artery pressures. The treatment is titrated continuously to a changing pressure or metabolic parameter. The future is here.

EMBRACING THE PATIENT LIFE CYCLE

In November 2003, a colleague asked me to see seventy-two-year-old Jim for a second opinion. Jim grew up in eastern Maine and had recently moved to the Boston area to seek medical care. He had been ill with failing kidneys for the seven years prior to seeing me. This had happened quite abruptly, after he developed a kidney infection that unfortunately progressed quite rapidly to both his kidneys losing their function. Jim had what some of us call the classic double whammy, severe heart and kidney failure. He had been written off. He was referred to me for his high risk of sudden death and the potential need for an implantable device that could shock his heart out of a fatal arrhythmia. Jim's heart function was less than a quarter of a normal heart. His left ventricular ejection fraction was 11 percent, with normal ejection fraction being anything above 50 percent. And he was on hemodialysis for failing kidneys. He was developing recurrent bouts of decompensated heart failure, for which he was repeatedly getting admitted to the hospital. Sometimes he would get readmitted within three days of being discharged. It was a no-win situation. It is particularly tough to manage a patient in this situation because they tend to retain fluid because of nonfunctioning kidneys and an inability to make urine, tipping them into heart failure. And sometimes an overzealous attempt to take off the excess fluid during dialysis can drop their blood pressure significantly, making the patient very symptomatic from that, too. Jim was not a candidate for a kidney transplant because of his exceedingly low heart function, and the consensus was that he would probably die on the table if doctors attempted anything invasive. When I met him, he was emaciated, had lost a lot of weight, and at six feet tall, weighed only 132 pounds. He was on a slippery slope to nowhere.

I noticed that he had some electrical-conduction abnormalities in his heart that could have been responsible for the poor contraction. This uncoordinated or dyssynchronous contraction within the heart is sometimes amenable to resynchronization by the placement of three wires in the heart to electrically pace the upper chamber (the right atrium) and both lower chambers (left and right ventricle). This therapy, known as cardiac resynchronization, was in its infancy two decades ago, and we were still trying to figure out who would respond to all this implantable hardware versus who would not. I decided to bite the bullet. What was there to lose? His clinical trajectory did not look good otherwise, with a projected lifespan of another three to six months at best. Despite the advice of some of my senior colleagues, I decided to take him up for the procedure. It was early days, and the technology was neither good nor robust enough, but after a six-hour-long procedure, I was able to suitably position the three wires in his heart. During the first couple of months post-implant, he continued to have a fairly tumultuous course, as his heart was getting used to a new way to contract. It was during this period that I conceived the idea for initiating a multidisciplinary clinic for these heart failure patients with implanted devices. These were very sick patients who needed to see an electrophysiologist, a heart failure specialist, and an imaging expert, among others. A multidisciplinary forum would serve as a one-stop shop for these patients, rather than the patient having to come on different days to see each of these specialists. It was the trekking back and forth from the hospital for several visits that often tipped these patients in the wrong direction. A simultaneous integrated visit seemed like a natural thing for Jim, who was exceedingly frail and could not make it to the hospital to see each of his consultants at their own specific times. He could barely walk ten steps before gasping for breath. Coming for each of those visits—waiting times plus driving in and out of the city—was enough to precipitate a heart failure episode.

Coupled with this, I felt that embracing these patients over their life cycle through their in- and outpatient phases via a coordinated care pathway, or what we now call a disease management platform using continuous digital data acquisition, would be revolutionary. The device companies were already ahead of the game and had begun providing us with stored data of the period between visits. This data was amazing and allowed us to get a sense of how the patient was doing over the several weeks before their appointment with us. This multidisciplinary clinic was well ahead of its time, as was the effort to put into place a remote-monitoring strategy. Through remote monitoring and repeated data downloads from the periods between the clinic visits, we were able to provide personalized care.

So what about Jim? Well, he did really well. His heart function improved over the next several months. His left ventricular ejection fraction at the end of the year was 64 percent, considered normal heart function. I was as surprised as he was. Interestingly, at the age of seventy-three, he became eligible for a renal transplant. His twenty-three-year-old neighbor from down the street donated her kidney to him. Another six months down the line, Jim was free of his heart and kidney failure. He was a changed man, with a new lease on life. He went on to become a dancing instructor at a senior center, where he met and married fifty-eight-year-old Donna. The two of them have been together for the last fourteen years. About eight years ago they moved to Florida, where Jim got back into the antique business. He recently turned ninety and is doing well. No more heart or kidney failure, though he has not managed to escape the other ills of growing old—multiple skin cancer surgeries, progressive deafness, and some vision loss. However, he continues to savor life. Jim has never forgotten that he was given a timeline of three months eighteen years ago.

4

THE SMARTWATCH ERA

I must govern the clock, not be governed by it.
GOLDA MEIR

I met Ned for the first time a few months ago at the urgent request of his primary care physician. Ned, a successful software engineer working at a local start-up, had become worried about experiencing recurrent episodes of a fast heartbeat, lasting for approximately fifteen seconds. Each time this occurred, it left him transiently light-headed. This brought back memories for him that made him afraid he might be having a stroke. Ned was thirty-nine years old, and he'd had a stroke six years prior. He had never had any medical problems and certainly no significant heart-related issues. There was no family history of a stroke, and the only relevant history was that of his father having mildly high blood pressure and some prediabetes, for which he was on medication and had made lifestyle changes. He had two siblings, an older sister and a younger brother, both, according to him, in immaculate health. They probably had not even ever seen a PCP, he said.

He recounted to me that six years ago, on a weekend morning, he was making breakfast for his kids, as he usually did. His wife usually slept in on the weekend, and he enjoyed doing his share of parenting in looking after their three- and five-year-old children, especially since it gave him some time to hang out and watch cartoons with them. He remembered distinctly that as he was reaching out for the cereal box, he felt strange, with a sudden weakness on his left side. He felt the carton slip from his hand, and he slumped to the kitchen floor with a thud. His wife immediately rushed to the kitchen on hearing the loud, awkward sound of his body hitting the floor and found him gazing in one direction, with garbled speech and the left side of his body limp. He remembered the EMTs arriving and being rushed to the hospital, where within the hour he completely recovered his speech and the strength in his arm.

The subsequent investigative workup in the hospital included an MRI of his brain, ECG monitoring, and an echocardiogram to look for any structural abnormality of his heart. The MRI showed that he'd had a small stroke, while the ECG monitoring didn't reveal any problems, and a transthoracic echocardiogram showed that he had a normal heart. His astute cardiologist at that time ordered a transesophageal echocardiogram, which involves placing the ultrasound probe down the throat into the esophagus to look more closely at the heart. This gives more direct access to the heart, allowing the cardiologist to look at the left atrium, the appendage, and the interatrial septum a little better than with a conventional echocardiogram, which is done from the outside by pressing the ultrasound probe to the outside of the chest.

During his echocardiogram, the imaging specialist injected a contrast agent to see whether there was a hole in the heart. Lo and behold, Ned had a PFO, which is short for a patent foramen ovale. This is a communication between the left and right atrium, representing a hole that is naturally present in our hearts before we are born to allow for the mixing of blood in both chambers, but as the heart evolves embryologically through our fetal life, it gets sealed off. In about 20 percent of patients, however, it doesn't. The risk with this is that a small percentage of patients can have a clot move from the right side of the body and heart directly to the left side, without getting filtered through the lungs. This can, in some circumstances, lead to a stroke, as it probably did in Ned. There was a lack of consensus among the specialists about whether the PFO was the true explanation for his symptoms and stroke, but after multiple opinions at leading academic centers across the city and beyond, Ned had his PFO closed by a simple interventional procedure using a two-sided clamp shell, which is placed across the interatrial septum, sealing it off and preventing any clot that develops in the venous system of the body from crossing over and going to the brain. Does this solve the problem, though?

On the day I saw him, he complained of palpitations, and after I probed a little, he said that he'd had palpitations and an irregular heart rate since his early teens. He had some of this around the time of his PFO closure, and now he was experiencing it again. Most notably, he had some very long episodes of palpitations after his PFO closure. This was diagnosed as atrial fibrillation and required an electrical shock to get him back in rhythm. He was also put on blood thinners at this time to help prevent his blood from forming a clot that could cause a stroke. When I asked him about his symptoms during childhood, Ned mentioned that he thought it was normal to have palpitations and his mother at one time had even taken him to see the school psychologist for what she thought was anxiety. But he was never told that he had a heart-rhythm disorder that could cause a stroke. He was never told that he had atrial fibrillation.

Could it be the PFO was a red herring and his main problem was actually atrial fibrillation, the most common heart-rhythm disturbance that also causes strokes? This is where medicine becomes murky. If there were a clear-cut way of temporally relating the stroke to a heart-rhythm issue through a sensor-based strategy, we would have been much closer to the truth, rather than making indirect inferences, as we are doing now. If medicine had a way of digitally tracking our heartbeat in a passive way through the course of our lives, thereby detecting atrial fibrillation or any other heart rhythm proactively, it could help preempt a life-threatening condition. Well, we can do that now. We just need to get better at it.

WATCHES AND ATRIAL FIBRILLATION

There are too many different types of smartwatches to list, though some common ones in the US include the Apple Watch, Garmin, Suunto 7, and Fitbit. Despite some differences, they all seek to measure the same physiological signals. There is a common interest among all of them toward identifying atrial fibrillation, which represents the commonest cardiac arrhythmia, affecting more than five million people in the United States. Atrial fibrillation increases the risk for a stroke by fivefold. It can also cause heart failure in a large percentage of patients by driving the heart rate very fast. A big concern is that this may be subclinical and mild and may go unnoticed until it becomes severe enough to manifest clinically, by which time it may be irreversible. It is noteworthy that atrial fibrillation without symptoms is associated with a similar risk of death, cardiovascular complications, or stroke, when compared to those who have symptoms during the initial manifestation. Not having symptoms does not mean that you are fine; in fact, to the contrary, that may lead to undetected progression. Smartwatches and other wearables can passively measure the pulse rate from the wrist. Wearable technology has the potential to flag health issues proactively, ensuring timely intervention. Most of these work via the same principle, using photoplethysmography (PPG), with an optical sensor that can measure the intermittency or the pulsatile nature of the blood flow in the wrist. This in turn enables the creation of a tachogram that is then analyzed by an algorithm, which can assess the regularity—or lack thereof—in these signals to help make the diagnosis of atrial fibrillation. An ECG app used in conjunction with the Fitbit Sense smartwatch allows the patient to take an ECG at any time. I recently interviewed Dr. Steven Lubitz, a professor at Harvard Medical School and the national principal investigator of the Fitbit Heart Study, which tested the PPG signal from the Fitbit watch in diagnosing atrial fibrillation in more than 455,000 patients. Although the watch worked well, with a positive predictive value in diagnosing atrial fibrillation of 98 percent, Steve did say that it is not all perfect. These watches, he said, worked best when the patient was inactive, to minimize disturbance in the recordings from motion and hand movement. This can have limitations when it comes to diagnosing the arrhythmia that may be brief and happens only during activity, which can be a common occurrence in some patients.

The recent Apple-sponsored Apple Heart Study was disruptive on many fronts. First, it bypassed the conventional patient-recruitment approach for a clinical trial, which usually involves a face-to-face consenting process. It used an app. All those patients needed was an Apple Watch, an iPhone, and a downloadable app. The Apple Heart Study was conducted as an observational trial in which 419,297 patients were enrolled to see whether the watch was useful in diagnosing atrial fibrillation. When the watch determined that five of six repeat tachograms suggested an irregular pulse, it set off a trigger of notification via the app to the participant in the study. The results showed that the watch was good, but not perfect, for diagnosing atrial fibrillation. The positive prediction value was lower than the Fitbit rate at 84 percent, and disconcerting to practicing clinicians, who feared being inundated by inquiries from patients who may be well but have a false-positive reading of atrial fibrillation from the watch. This could overwhelm the hospital systems and at the same time invoke a fear factor among patients. A watch with the ability to diagnose an arrhythmia is a double-edged sword: on one hand it can help disseminate a diagnostic tool across the population, but at the same time, its diagnosing ability is not on par with conventional shorter-duration noninvasive diagnostic tools such as the ECG, the patch monitor, Holter monitor, or implantable devices such as the loop recorder.

Detecting atrial fibrillation (A-fib) accurately is a big deal, especially because of the high prevalence and increasing incidence of this condition. The projections are that with an aging population, the changing demographics will increase the number of atrial fibrillation patients to twelve million by 2050. So if even a small fraction of patients were false positives as detected by the watch, one can only imagine the horrendous and overwhelming workload this may impose on a practicing clinician. On the other hand, I am quite sure that over time, the fidelity of the signals will improve, as will the algorithms for further enhancing the positive predictive value of these tracings. Many companies in the AI space, such as Cardiologs, are developing cloud-based approaches to enhance algorithms to make this strategy automatic, reliable, deployable, and scalable. There is also considerable work happening in the role of neural networks toward predicting cardiac function, mortality, and arrhythmias from a simple, short smartwatch ECG strip. Imagine a tool like a watch that can not only pinpoint heart-rhythm disturbances in real time but can warn you of ominous events in the near future. A new age has dawned.

CONTRADICTIONS AND CONTROVERSIES

Not everyone is a fan of the role of the smartwatch in diagnosing atrial fibrillation. In fact, Milton Packer, a cardiologist of national repute, called it a serious competitor for the worst heart device ever. In his blog he stated that this could put the general community on hyperalert and make them more anxious than they need to be. Most of the people in the Apple Heart Study were under forty, approximating almost 220,000 individuals. Among these only 341 (16 percent) patients were informed of an irregularity in their rhythm; of those, only nine (.4 percent) actually had atrial fibrillation. And to quote him further, "Overall the chances of the Apple watch detecting undiagnosed atrial fibrillation in this study were lower than the chance of a person being struck by lightning during their lifetime (0.03 percent)."

There is certainly an element of truth to its lack of immediate clinical applicability. At this stage it is proof of concept, but many questions remain unanswered about A-fib that would make the indiscriminate use of this technology to diagnose and detect A-fib rather cumbersome. We have no idea of the risk for death, stroke, or cardiovascular events in patients who have A-fib first detected by a smartwatch. Can we prevent death or stroke, or is there a role for blood thinners to prevent strokes in smartwatch-detected A-fib? There is always the potential for this device to falsely alert healthy individuals and create anxiety. Before encouraging widespread use, we need a better understanding of the knowledge gained from a PPG-guided tachogram that suggests the presence of atrial fibrillation.

Leadership within Apple is overly optimistic on the role of the Apple Watch, and Apple's COO, Jeff Williams, has stated that the watch will be the ultimate guardian of users' health. This is still far from being realized. The recent addition of the oxygen saturation sensor to the Apple watch is a step in the right direction. Some of the answers to the many posed questions lie in executing a definitive trial to prove the worth of this monitoring system. This would need to be randomized and have hard clinical endpoints that the clinicians could hang their hats on. The study will need to have a large cohort of individuals across all age-groups, where everyone in the trial will get a watch but only half the participants will receive information from the watch. And, of course, the study will need to be adequately powered with large numbers of patients to see whether the intervention reduces the risk of stroke and death.

Kim Eagle, editor in chief of the website for the American College of Cardiology (ACC.org), was quoted as saying that "the accuracy of the watch is still short of more traditional and currently used techniques. This is just a glimpse of the future, but we have a ways to go."

This is important, because with the increasing incidence of A-fib, there is also the increased risk for morbidity. A-fib increases the risk of a stroke by fivefold and can be asymptomatic and subclinical in many patients. Almost a quarter of patients I see with A-fib do not have symptoms. It is often detected accidentally during a routine examination, or the patient may present for the first time not with palpitations, but with symptoms of shortness of breath from a failing heart. A fast heart rate from A-fib that has gone undetected for several weeks can fatigue the heart muscle, resulting in heart failure. In a significant number of A-fib patients, a stroke may be the first presenting symptom. Also noteworthy is that one-fifth of all the strokes related to A-fib, the stroke may in fact be the initial presentation of atrial fibrillation.

It makes sense to have a population-based screening strategy, since we know that four-fifths of the population have smartphones, and nearly 15 percent of those wear smartwatches. The role of the watch in A-fib is still up in the air, based on some of the reservations pertinent to the maturity of the technology. It may have a better role in a preselected, enriched population with already established atrial fibrillation, where we are looking for recurrences of A-fib to decide on a form of therapy. Also, monitoring of heart failure patients may be useful, since when they develop A-fib, their prognosis can become markedly worse.

It is unclear what the role or impact of this wearable technology will be on low-risk young patients with highly transient asymptomatic A-fib. The question of whether this form of subclinical disease is clinically meaningful is up for debate. Some key opinion leaders feel that in the absence of other risk factors (e.g., diabetes, hypertension, age over sixty-five years, or vascular disease), there is nothing to worry about. Interestingly, 3 percent of the population over sixty-five years have asymptomatic atrial fibrillation, and this in turn could have significant public health implications. On the flip side, others (me included) are of the opinion that subclinical transient A-fib may be a harbinger for future A-fib. It is akin to prediabetes, which develops into full diabetes in most patients. If the right lifestyle modification measures are put into place, then like adult-onset diabetes, atrial fibrillation may also be completely preventable.

But the magic of the smartwatch does not stop here. It can for certain modify the way we look at routine and emergent care. The well-publicized *Boston Globe* story of Dan Pfau, a seventy-year-old retired management consultant, comes to mind. While biking on Martha's Vineyard, Dan maneuvered off the bike path onto a less-traveled, unpaved trail. He hit a bump that knocked him off his bike, and the next thing he remembers is being in an ambulance. He does not remember phoning for help, but the watch automatically did so. The sensor in the Apple Watch can detect a fall, and if the user does not move for sixty seconds, the watch automatically puts a call in for assistance. In the ER, Dan was noted to have a brain hemorrhage, for which he was helicoptered to Mass General Hospital in Boston for further care. The speed with which the Apple watch intervened certainly helped prevent what could have been a tough situation. As I have often stated in my lectures, we need to "watch out for watches, because soon the watch will be watching out for us."

WATCHES, APPS, AND RESEARCH STUDIES

The Apple Heart and Fitbit Heart studies have revolutionized the way we conduct clinical trials. Both these studies used remote strategies for recruitment, consenting, follow-up, and management of the study participants. Although both studies could be criticized for either lack of outcomes or a modest number of false positives, it depends on what lens you are wearing while interpreting these studies. They were both large, ambitious studies that showed that the watch can be used to detect atrial fibrillation; however, further refinement is still necessary.

Using an app for study recruitment is certainly something that many of us have been discussing for a while, and it is terrific to see this launched at a population level. This will significantly democratize how research is done and enable the generation of large datasets that will in turn change the playing field. It will be interesting to see how this will be integrated into electronic medical records (EMRs) in the future, as that is what will truly determine the clinical value and utility. Having wearables that are seamlessly integrated into daily living will enable behavioral modification that could be shown to positively influence disease states and outcomes. Showing the impact of mobility and heart rate at a population level would be meaningful in many ways, not only by reducing costs through simpler lifestyle strategies but also by promoting overall wellness. Watches for surveillance, risk stratification, diagnosis of specific disease states, and facilitating lifestyle interventions will be an important part of our arsenal in combating sickness.

WATCHES, COVID, AND FUTURE PANDEMICS?

The pandemic certainly brought to the forefront the need for a digital infrastructure and remote patient-monitoring services. In my experience of following nine patients with implantable devices who developed COVID, sensor-based data could pick up changes prior to the patient experiencing symptoms. We were able to off-load the digital data from their implanted devices for weeks prior to them contracting COVID and then for several weeks during and after their recovery. An elevated heart rate, reduction in physical activity, and changes in lung impedance (due to COVID pneumonia) closely correlated with the patients' symptoms and predated the hospitalization. These measures normalized in a few days after discharge from the hospital. Wearable technology and smartwatches can provide the same and even more information.

Many watch-derived metrics such as heart rate, heart rate variability, respiration rate, activity, sleep, and oxygen saturations that can now be used to monitor patients with heart disease and failure can also serve to pick up early infections as well as monitor patients during the entire affliction. Elevation of the heart rate is a direct consequence of the fever. It is the body's effort to mount a defense response to the virus. Heart rate variability, as described earlier, is a reflector of overall health and stress. A lower heart rate variability is associated with a worse outcome and, in patients with cardiac disease, is associated with increased mortality. COVID-19 can stress the cardiovascular system by releasing adrenaline that increases the resting heart rate and average overall heart rate and can affect blood pressure. Sleep can be detected via measurements of the heart rate and accelerometer data, which can be used to quantify the duration and quality of sleep. An increased sleep duration coupled with poor-quality sleep has been shown to occur in COVID-19 patients.

The beauty of these wearables is the simplicity. They can be useful at both the population and individual level. At the population level, they can help identify communities at risk while monitoring the spread of disease and objectively quantifying the impact of a public health intervention on a broad scale. Using machine learning, one can reliably detect and measure population health status, which can help stave off surges and other scourges. At the individual level, smartwatches have found a place in the real-time detection of COVID-19. They can detect changes in physiology prior to the development of symptoms. There are ways for the smartwatch to identify a deviation from the baseline (through changes in heart rate, physical activity, oxygen saturations, and so on) with a multitiered alarm strategy to prevent false positives. This allows patients to begin self-isolation proactively before clinical confirmation of the illness. This also allows the watch to monitor disease progression at home, as well as in the hospital. Remote monitoring of these devices enables early detection and the appropriate escalation of care at home. Also, quickly and objectively identifying the need for transfer to a hospital environment for closer monitoring and care is of paramount importance.

Almost 20 percent of the population have smartwatches, and anonymized data pulled from the cloud and localized to zip codes and neighborhoods could provide public health officials and researchers a valuable tool to pinpoint areas at increased risk for infections and spread. However, there remains much ground to cover on several issues: data privacy and data sharing, adherence to monitoring, impact of social disparities, and gaps in the equity of care. The overlap in the use of smartwatches between the average healthy consumer and the patient provides a huge opportunity for early detection and prevention of disease. The work has only just begun.

5

CONTINUOUS CARE AND NOVEL SENSORS: A RECIPE FOR HEALTH

Health is not valued till sickness comes.
THOMAS FULLER

I remember the date clearly. It was January 29, 2019, when I got a call from my PCP. Dr. Tso told me in a very concerned tone that my hemoglobin A1C (HbA1c) was 10.5. I have learned over the years that the HbA1c is a much better measure of diabetes than an episodic fasting blood glucose check. As a blood test it measures the cumulative exposure of the body to elevated blood sugar levels over a six-week period. It tells you whether your blood glucose levels have been consistently elevated, as opposed to high just one time. The normal A1C level is supposed to be less than 6.0; anything above that suggests it may be time to begin paying attention to what you eat and how much you exercise, because your body is not metabolizing glucose well enough.

Clearly mine was not. It was elevated to a level that I thought I might need to take insulin. I was stunned, as I had always looked after myself and presumed I was healthy. But then thinking back, we had just moved (I hear it is comparable to the physical stress of labor), I had stopped exercising, and much of my day was tied up between clinical and administrative work. Lunch was episodic, and cookies and vending machines were often easily accessible. So clearly, there was an explanation. Nevertheless, I was shocked. Especially since less than a year prior, my HbA1c was 6.2. I immediately sought guidance from the endocrinology group at my hospital. We figured out very quickly that I needed to change my diet, begin exercising, and lose a little bit of weight in addition to commencing metformin.

I was armed with glucose strips to check my blood sugar daily. I quickly realized that I needed some feedback beyond the periodic stick in the finger. This was better than nothing, but not particularly user-friendly. Each time you wanted to know your blood glucose, it meant pricking your finger with a lancet and analyzing the drop of blood with a sensor device to read out your blood glucose level. This was kind of painful, especially if you tend to bruise easily and need to use your hands for doing invasive procedures and surgeries. Beyond this, it did not tell me what foods were affecting me in what way, so that I could modify and adapt my behavior accordingly. That's when I found out about continuous glucose monitoring using a blood glucose sensor (FreeStyle Libre). This is a wearable device with a little sensor that is positioned on the underside of the arm. One could also call it semi-implantable, since a part of the sensor pin punctures your skin and sits in the tissue just below the skin. It can be self-implanted in a painless and user-friendly way. Then, using your phone and the app, you can scan the sensor to find out your blood glucose in real time at any time. This sensor measures glucose and stores readings throughout the day. Every day was a teaching moment for me to learn how my blood glucose level fluctuated with the time of the day, drinking coffee, exercising, enjoying a glass of wine, and eating. I could figure out which foods caused my blood glucose levels to fluctuate. Contrary to conventional beliefs, there were foodstuffs that I thought were good for me, such as oatmeal, that would result in high blood sugar levels. I know that is not the case for everyone, with or without diabetes. The feedback was phenomenal and allowed me to modify my lifestyle and get back in normal range in less than four months. One year later, I was down to an A1C of 5.9 on the lowest possible dose of metformin, and two years later, I was off medications.

CONTINUOUS CARE

Diabetes is a chronic disease that affects more than thirty million people in the United States alone. The condition, associated with an abnormal metabolism of blood glucose, occurs when the pancreas is unable to adjust insulin levels to help keep blood glucose levels in check. In type 2 diabetes, similar to what I have, the problem is often a resistance to insulin, where the pancreas cannot keep pace with the demand and the glucose levels rise and remain high for extended periods of time. Elevated glucose levels can have terrible downstream effects. They can damage almost any organ in the body, including the kidneys, brain, heart, and nerves. They can even damage the blood vessels in any part of the body. Kidney failure, heart attacks, sudden death, and blindness are well-known long-term complications of uncontrolled diabetes. When you speak to some diabetics, you will sense a great deal of frustration with the daily struggle of trying to get ahead of their disease. Much of the care is reactive, and as alluded to before, blood sugar levels often vacillate unpredictably. There is enough evidence to suggest that more frequent testing is associated with better control and outcomes. The more you test, the better your ability to adapt your lifestyle and medication in an educated way.

In an attempt to monitor glucose levels, a spectrum of potential sensors has evolved over the years. These could include measures beyond the conventional finger-stick method that most diabetics get used to performing multiple times a day. This could be a subcutaneous sensor, such as the FreeStyle Libre or the Dexcom G6, which is implanted below the skin, or an ocular sensor in the form of a contact lens (e.g., Google or Verily Life Sciences), which can monitor glucose levels in tears. This gives a readout with the help of a handheld device or smartphone. There are watch sensors that produce small electric shocks to open up the pores and extract fluid to monitor tissue glucose concentrations. Sensor-laden toilets can provide readouts of urinary glucose levels that can be automatically transmitted to provider offices wirelessly. One can speculate that, in the future, disease-specific smart sensors will be linked to an implanted drug reservoir. This could be insulin for a diabetic, or a sensor for the appropriate drug for viral count in a patient with HIV, or an antihypertensive agent for a sustained elevation in blood pressure. Recently Welldoc obtained FDA approval for its BlueStar diabetes management solutions. The insulin-adjustment program from BlueStar allows care as and when the patient needs it, which prevents doctors from having to spend time poring over the minutiae of dose adjustment so they can instead concentrate on other more practical and intellectual elements of patient care.

Most current wearables and sensors are used for general fitness and wellness purposes. But many other daily activities can influence health. One of these is sleep. We spend one-third of our life sleeping, and it will not surprise anyone that abnormal sleep patterns are associated with disease.

This can be a cause and effect, where sleep abnormalities can cause heart disease and vice versa. Teasing out the chicken-and-egg relationship is sometimes instrumental in deciding what to treat, the sleep issue or the heart disease, or both. There are several sensors that help monitor sleep rhythm and oxygen saturations. Sleep apnea is a common clinical disorder where the individual has periods of apnea—stops breathing for a few seconds—followed by a period of hyperventilation. It is a problem that has many secondary ill effects, like the development of heart-rhythm issues and narcolepsy, which is characterized by excessive sleepiness and lack of energy during the day. Notably, sleep apnea is usually associated with a high body mass index. There are FDA-approved oral devices such as the DentiTrac, which is prescribed for sleep apnea. This device contains sensors that can monitor temperature, head position, and movement. Beyond this, the smartphone itself and a wearable hand device can monitor oxygen saturations as well as sleep patterns and assist with the diagnosis of sleep apnea. This form of continuous monitoring is more than a snapshot. The data trends reflect how both good days and bad days look. Care is then individualized per person and, in time, continuously.

Other forms of continuous wearable monitoring include the Vega GPS tracker, a wearable sensor for ensuring safety for people with Alzheimer's disease. This helps in monitoring the location of the patient via the use of GPS. Some wristbands for epilepsy (Empatica) can monitor physiological signals in epileptic people and alert family in real time about an impending seizure. Other sensors used in areas where malaria is endemic include a bracelet for monitoring temperature and sweat patterns in children, with alerts sent to parents' smartphones to apprise them of data suggestive of malaria. Wearable UV sensors in the form of a bracelet, armband, or wristband can warn us about excessive and harmful UV exposure, which can cause skin aging, burns, and skin cancer. Stress is an everyday trigger for illness. Sensors that measure heart rate, its variability, and sweat patterns can help gauge the level of the autonomic tone and ensuing stress. Sensor-driven alerts designed with a nudge to break free from the inciting trigger and disrupt a vicious cycle will serve as a great recipe for health. Optical fiber sensors within bed mattresses can provide noncontact monitoring of respiratory rate and heart rate during sleep—a low-cost, daily-use long-term home-monitoring solution for patients with sleep apnea or lung or heart diseases. Many of these sensors and their signals are still being refined as they gradually become a part of the daily workflow of monitoring.

CARING ACROSS BORDERS

A few years ago, one of my patients, a US federal agent posted in the eastern European bloc, developed atrial fibrillation. He spent at least nine months a year out of the country and saw me on a yearly basis when he was back in the US. Doug was thirty-four years old when he developed atrial fibrillation (A-fib). It was discovered accidentally when he developed symptoms of shortness of breath due to a very fast heart rate from his A-fib. It is worth mentioning that approximately one-fourth of the patients who have A-fib may not feel it. They do not notice any symptoms of a racing heart. In fact, they come to our attention when they develop overt signs of either heart failure or present with sudden-onset paralysis from a stroke. The heart begins to fail from the stress of beating at high rates for several days and weeks under the radar, without the patient's knowledge. On the other hand, a fibrillating atrium can lead to the development of a clot in the left atrium, which may then get dislodged and cut off circulation in a part of the brain, causing a stroke.

After Doug was diagnosed with A-fib, I cardioverted him back into normal rhythm. This involves delivering an electric shock to the chest that helps jump-start or reboot the heart, a routine procedure for many patients when they first manifest with persistent forms of atrial fibrillation that do not automatically go away. I then started him on an anti-arrhythmic medication called flecainide, which changes the electrical properties of the atrial musculature and helps hold patients in normal sinus rhythm. As good as these drugs are, they are not foolproof. In fact, their success rate of holding a patient consistently in normal rhythm is about 60 percent over the course of a year. So, obviously, Doug was worried. One, because he lived many thousands of miles away, and also because he did not feel his A-fib and was not sure when he was going in and out of it. He was worried that a recurrence would go unnoticed and he would present in heart failure again. He was too young to have recurrent bouts of heart failure. That's when we embarked on using a sensor-based approach to monitor his A-fib from a distance. We settled on trying AliveCor (with the Kardia app), a sensor-based approach that could be attached to a smartphone. All it required was for the patient to download the app, then place his thumbs on the sensor pads to generate an ECG. This could then be transmitted electronically as a PDF to the clinician, or one could access this through the patient's portal with their permission. At the time of writing this, there is still no clear, uniform approach to integrate this with our electronic medical record system . . . but it should happen soon.

This turned out to work exceedingly well. Doug had a few recurrences in Romania that we were able to treat over the phone with extra doses of his medicine. He eventually had a catheter ablation of his A-fib as a curative strategy. It was evident from his imaging and recordings from his heart during the invasive procedure that Doug had experienced occasional A-fib episodes for a long time, though it had remained below the radar for several years. His atrium was enlarged but also showed areas of remodeling and scarring, something that only happens over time. The ablation was successful, and Doug has been free of A-fib for several years. He has moved on from Eastern Europe to Southeast Asia. He still sends me transmissions to make sure everything is in sync. Most recently he sent me a transmission (a PDF of his rhythm) from his honeymoon in the Maldives. I am presuming it was good for him to be reassured that he did not have A-fib then.

THE CHALLENGE OF TOO MUCH

As good as this sounds in anecdotal cases, the integration of wearables into one's practice is not without logistical hurdles. One can only imagine the thousands of patients in the Rolodex sending transmissions to the clinic willy-nilly any time they feel slightly off-center; however, that is the future. There is no going backward. The patient is the point of care. We expect immediate care or attention for a symptom that is bothering us. It may seem trivial to others, but the moment it is *us*, the relative importance of any symptom changes. You need attention . . . and now! The problem can be gradual indication creep. First, transmissions may be specific, but then they can be for marginal symptoms, a manifestation of a curiosity factor. *Hmm, I feel tired, so let me see if my heart rate or temperature is out of whack*, and if even a tad off-center, one can imagine a whole cadre of patients looking for reassurance from their physician that they don't have any life-threatening condition incipiently creeping up on them. On the other hand, stable measures could be reassuring and prevent an unwarranted visit to or contact with the clinic. It is a two-edged sword. There will need to be careful education and individualized alert strategies.

SENSORS FOR ALL BY 2030

Sensors are everywhere—in us, on us, and outside of us. Advances in technology have allowed for the development of a variety of sensors that can enable the monitoring of a slew of physiological signals. As stated earlier, many of these capabilities now lie within our smartphones, and these phones are disseminated to more than five billion people across the world. The extension of wireless networks into rural and low-income areas provides us with the prospect of fulfilling the motto of "Health for all." The ubiquitous presence of wireless networks coupled with the future availability of wearable and implantable devices and sensors to monitor and deliver health care in remote areas can change the dynamics. There is now a low-cost option for providing access to health care for the underprivileged and aging populations. We are in a position to dispense low-cost sensors that will change the face of health care delivery.

We need to recognize that and begin to embrace it. The goal is to provide care wherever the patient may be, and at whatever time. Simplistically, it is the integration of information technology and health care to provide care for the diagnosis, prevention, treatment, and follow-up of the patient. This represents the fourth industrial revolution, a convergence of science and technology that involves superintelligence and hyperconnectivity. The synergy between the internet of things (IoT), cloud computing, and Big-Data technologies along with the continually evolving forms of mobile health (mHealth) and virtual care will comprise smart health.

The smartphone, wearables, implantables, and other sensors in the environment together create the IoT. The IoT component will allow different devices to collect and exchange data in an automated way. This will enable hospitals and caregivers to seamlessly connect with virtual assistants at home, exchanging information regarding blood pressure, heart rate, temperature, oxygen saturations, and so on, facilitating the provision of preventative care and appropriately timed treatment. This is particularly important when we are treating patients who can decompensate rather quickly, be it a patient with asthma, thyroid disease, Parkinson's disease, heart failure, or brittle diabetes. The sensors of the future will cater to the overall well-being of the population, be disease specific, and be remarkably patient-centric.

BIOSENSORS, INGESTIBLE, AND TOUCH SENSORS

Biosensors will be noninvasive in most instances, passively providing information to either the patient or the monitoring setup, depending on the underlying disease state and the extent of monitoring required. The use of alternative analytes besides finger sticks will include the potential role of tears, saliva, sweat, urine, and exhaled breaths. There are already many smartphone-based approaches to using colorimetric data, which can be converted to digital images. There are disposable paper-plastic hybrid microfluidic devices for such analysis on urine, to report on pH, glucose, or red blood cells. This in turn can allow patients to expedite these measurements at home, without a visit to the doctor.

As discussed earlier, perspiration sensors provide real-time measurements of electrolyte status of a patient. This could include sodium, potassium, trace minerals, and even other metabolites like lactate and glucose. These can provide direct evidence of the disease state, assess risk for drug interactions, and assist with wellness approaches. IoT-embedded sweat-monitoring systems can send information directly to the smartphone, which could be integrated with the patient's EMR or the cloud. Miniaturization, flexible electronics, and advances in biosensor technology have made this possible.

Nonadherence to medications is a critical problem in the management of patients. There are many reasons for this, but the real issue is that this is known to occur across different disease states and medications and directly affects clinical outcomes. When this behavior is put into the equation of chronic diseases, where it occurs the most, there is a colossal loss of money. Poor adherence accentuates health care expenditure and accounts for roughly $100 to $300 billion in unnecessary medical costs in the US alone. This is a serious medical problem that affects patients, health planners, policy makers, payers, and physicians. It is not new, and there have been many mitigation strategies for this over the years based on self-reporting, pill counts, or prescription refill histories. Unfortunately, all these are generally inaccurate and incomplete and seem inappropriate for precisely measuring drug adherence. There are many contributing factors to nonadherence, of which forgetfulness is the commonest explanation.

Newer, ingestible event-monitoring systems (such as the ID-Cap system) can help detect an ingested drug from the GI tract. This comprises a microsensor embedded in an oral pill and activated by stomach juices. The sensor communicates digital messages to an external wearable reader (patch), confirming ingestion of the drug. These data, inclusive of a time-stamped message confirming ingestion, are transmitted to a secure central remote-monitoring system. The patch also measures activity, heart rate, and step count. The app engages the patients with nonpharmacological therapies, physical activity, feedback on taking medication, and prompts to remind them about taking their medications.

When it comes to thinking about the evolution of sensors and their integration into day-to-day future care, we overlook touch as a sense. Touch is very complicated. The measuring of finger-pad skin displacement allows us to perceive the direction of a tactile experience. It is understandable that robotic prostheses and limb replacements will need a high level of dexterity if we are looking to equate the experience of a natural and normal hand or foot. Even though the development of artificial tactile sensors that are deformable and can perceive the same level of touch directionality is possible, there is a greater complexity that needs the assistance of AI. This requires convolutional neural networks to help develop an experience over a range of angles and speed of deformation and grasps. And then we have artificial stretchy skin that can be connected to our nervous system and can make amputees feel again. Equally fascinating is the development of a bionic hand with vision sensors that see an object and direct the hand toward the object to grasp it.

DISEASE-SPECIFIC SENSORS

Sensimed (Lausanne, Switzerland) recently received clearance for its Triggerfish contact lens, embedded with microsensors that can track the progression of glaucoma. This disposable lens continuously records spontaneous ocular dimensional changes that are transmitted to a recorder, which then is transmitted to the physician's computer via Bluetooth. Although there have been some glitches in the smart contact lenses impregnated with glucose sensors, the use of wireless power transfer circuits and LED pixels allows the constant monitoring of glucose levels in tears. The issue, however, has been the correlation of these measurements with blood glucose levels. Could this be a new parameter used for diabetes control, with the definition of a new normal with measurements made in analytes other than blood? Using alternative analytes to blood may mean redefining new normal values for the population and, importantly, for the patient, so that early deviations can be quickly detected.

Asthma is a common clinical condition accounting for a large proportion of emergency room visits in pediatric and adult hospitals. There are innovations such as the ADAMM device, delivering Intelligent Asthma Management, which has a soft, flexible, waterproof, wearable IoT that connects and communicates via Wi-Fi and Bluetooth connections with both smartphone apps and a web-based portal. This hypoallergenic, skin-safe adhesive can pick up early symptoms that may indicate the potential for an asthma flare, thereby allowing early detection and intervention. The surrogates for a flare are simple and measure respiratory rate and patterns, cough rate, temperature, and heart rate. This data can be compared with the patient's prior patterns or reach a trigger point that can be used as an objective parameter for intervention. This is especially useful in younger and older patients who find it difficult to communicate early symptoms of their discomfiture. Other examples of IoT-enabled devices include those that allow blood glucose monitoring through a dongle, such as iBGStar, which transfers the data to a cloud server that physicians can access via the web.

Epilepsy is another unpredictable and scary condition. Besides the generalized tonic-clonic seizures, epilepsy can also be associated with sudden death. Seizures can now be detected by wearable devices and sensors embedded in a bed. These can trigger alarms, prompting immediate intervention by caregivers, leading to a decreased risk of sudden death. Other sensors in the epileptic patient can provide complementary information such as postseizure oxygen saturations, electrocardiograms, autonomic dysfunction, heart rate, and ectodermal activity, all of which could serve as markers of the postseizure clinical state.

LIFE, LIVING, AND SENSORS

The potential of virtual-assist strategies for daily disease management is quite limitless, specifically, for diseases that have measurable parameters that need to be monitored. We know that atrial fibrillation can be measured and detected by changes in heart rate and irregularity, while diabetes is tracked by blood glucose, and blood pressure provides objective measures of how well hypertension is being treated. Now imagine that this, along with weight, oxygen saturations, respiratory rate, voice tone, and so on, can all be linked to your Alexa or any personal virtual-assist device that is powered by commonly available simpler forms of AI that use natural language processing. This would not only log and tabulate your readings but could serve to remind, nudge, or provide repeated educational instructions.

This is all happening in real time. Alexa has the ability to transmit data. In fact, a company called Livongo allows members to use the device to query their last blood sugar trends and receive insights and prods that are personalized to them. This form of virtual assistance will help provide the personalized care that we lack today in care delivery. Virtual doc visits paired with a prior understanding of the overall health status through a perusal of the electronic health records will take preventative care to the next level. Companies like Kinetxx can provide patients with virtual physical therapy without the patient even having to go to the gym—all within the comfort of one's own home. The real question is how the business model will work. Will these be out of pocket or strategies supported by health insurance companies? This is discussed at greater length in Part IV: Future Models of Care.

What use is sensing if there is no action to follow? What use is an action if it cannot be backed by the highest level of intelligence and simulate the ultimate human experience? Look at something as simple as blinking—it is a complex reflex involving the brain. A slew of medical conditions can affect the eyelids and cause eyelid muscle spasms. This is known as blepharospasm, defined as involuntary closure of the eyelids due to spasms of the orbicularis oculi muscle that surrounds the eyes and interdigitates into the eyelid. There are new soft nanomembrane sensors embedded with flexible hybrid bioelectronics under development. These are conformable and can gently laminate the skin around the eyes while enabling wireless quantitative electrophysiological signals that can measure the clinical symptoms, frequency of blinking, and spasms of the eye muscle that lead to eye closures. Now, as simple as this may sound, it requires deep learning and a convolutional network with the bioelectronic signals to enable the real-time classification of key pathological features and construct an effector response to mitigate the symptoms. As good as sensors may be at changing the paradigm, their impact is incomplete and, in some cases, inconsequential without the integration of AI-based strategies to complete the circuit of delivering care. More of this is discussed in Part III, Chapter 13 and 14.

FEEDBACK AND THE CARE CONTINUUM

Feedback is one of the best ways for patients to take charge of their health. Just as a blood glucose sensor tells you which foodstuffs cause your blood sugar to spike, the same applies to a variety of other diseases and conditions (e.g., heart failure, asthma, allergies, or lupus). As regards atrial fibrillation, certain activities, or consumables such as wine, caffeine, chocolate, and cheese, among others, can trigger it. It is not an all-or-nothing phenomenon. Some patients can have six cups of coffee a day and never trigger their A-fib, but one glass of red wine can tip them into an intractable episode or make them experience skipped beats. It is a question of individual susceptibility that we clearly don't have an exact explanation for. But wearables with an immediate feedback strategy can help us modify our lifestyle and make some choices that can attenuate or prevent disease flare-ups.

Gregory Marcus, professor of the School of Medicine at the University of California, San Francisco, has pioneered studies in the arena of wearables and trigger-testing. When speaking with Greg, I learned these are complicated studies that require active participation and interest by the patients to help find and isolate the triggers responsible for their symptoms. These are called N of 1 trials, which most agree is the purest form of a clinical study, where the impact of an intervention is evaluated in the same subject. Here patients serve as their own control subjects while testing the impact of each trigger (e.g., alcohol or caffeine) to incite atrial fibrillation. Studies that were previously thought to be logistically challenging can now be done more easily with wearable strategies, smartwatches, and apps that provide immediate feedback. Professor Marcus showed that among all triggers, alcohol was the only consistent provocative trigger for atrial fibrillation. Go figure!

A patient's need for speedy reassurance through direct instant contact with the clinical team is often underestimated. Wearables provide that. The presence of a wearable and the determination of the underlying rhythm obviate the need for a patient to get away from work and travel many miles to get to the clinic for an ECG—and the ECG may well be normal by the time the patient gets to the hospital. Also, the patient may feel well by then, so we have a futile visit, with time expended on both ends with an added cost to the health system. We forget taking into consideration the cost to the patient in terms of leaving their job, traveling, maneuvering through traffic, and parking, all of which can take up the better part of a day, sometimes for absolutely nothing.

CHALLENGES AND SOLUTIONS

On the other hand, the use of wearables may deprive the health system of the generation of some revenue through a copayment, an ECG, and usually additional (often unnecessary) laboratory testing. As silly as that may sound, there are hospitals and practices clinging to every possible revenue-generating strategy, although from a broader perspective, it is quite apparent that this truly is unwarranted. We are all talking about value-based care, and it is time to put our money where our mouth is, as there is nothing more valuable than expediency, eliminating redundancy, and enhancing the patient experience. The health care system is broken, and preserving its viability and mission are discussed at length in Part IV of this book. If one can reassure the patient from a distance that all is well and there is no need for them to come all the way in, that is time well spent.

However, it doesn't stop there. There is a slew of wearables, and every patient comes in with a different device that measures different variables in different ways. Some of them are trying to measure the same thing, but in dissimilar ways. Some watches just measure heart rate irregularity. Is the rhythm regular or irregular? If it happens to be irregular, then you have A-fib. These devices don't have ECG rhythm strips to back up the irregularity, which makes it challenging in many ways. For one, we know many forms of heart-rhythm disturbances can cause irregular pulses that may not be A-fib. These could be extra beats coming from the lower or upper chambers of the heart. The treatment and urgency of care for each of these conditions vary widely among patients. So for a system to get immediately integrated with one's clinic flow, there needs to be a validated tool that shows some objectivity to the measure. Also, the devices need to be FDA approved if one is going to make clinical decisions from them.

Some practices have this figured out. They have a lawyer-approved one-page document that spells out the dos, don'ts, and expectations for patients. The patients send in their AliveCor ECG recordings, which are downloaded on a weekly basis, and the results are sent back to them in a week's time. The patients are forewarned by the participating physicians that if they are having symptoms, they need to call the clinic offices. Integrating this into the workflow is important. In this practice, patients get the AliveCor device, sign the consent form, and enroll with the service that allows the physicians access to the patient portal. That way, no transmissions need to be made and the clinic service accesses the site weekly to make sure that nothing is amiss.

It will not be long before the watches come up with their own application interface with the EMR. There are ongoing endeavors using the Apple HealthKit (iPhone app) to enable the export of an ECG that could be integrated with the EMR, and Amazon Halo already has made limited inroads into EMR integration. The autonomous reading of these ECG signals using AI algorithms is currently being validated, refined, and deployed. As discussed in the AI section, sophisticated readouts from these tracings will be able to provide information beyond just heart rhythm and rate. Deep-learning tools will prognosticate and risk-stratify patients for future cardiac events, death, and strokes.

Finding the sweet spot of transmissions, workload, and reimbursement and assessing the place they have in value-based care is still a work in progress. Nevertheless, these technologies remain a good way of monitoring patients after starting a new medication or after a catheter ablation. Studies like the BOAT OAR study (Better Outcomes for Anticoagulation Treatment through Observation of Atrial Rhythm) specifically examine whether patients with a smartphone are more likely to use blood thinners if they are using an A-fib monitoring system. Sometimes, the mind doesn't comprehend what the eye can't see, especially when you feel well. Being faced with data (e.g., an abnormal ECG, blood pressure, or oxygen saturations) that speaks to the contrary can change that. The downstream impact of how we treat any disorder will be deeply affected by this data. How much of medical therapy must be episodic, versus continuous, on a daily basis remains to be determined.

Then there is the new-toy phenomenon, which worries most clinicians. The data overload makes us fearful. There is the hope that we will be forced to find a way to integrate this seamlessly into the workflow that does not overload staff but at the same time provides real-time care, enhancing the patient experience. Just like home-based blood pressure cuffs and blood glucose monitoring, there was much trepidation in promoting self-management, but I think these anxieties were overstated. Patients are quick learners and now use these systems all the time. It is refreshing to have a patient come in with their blood pressure and blood glucose nicely charted, so you can see the circadian variation and not just the single in-office measurement that was out of the norm. This will expand to all these new wearables, and we must not be afraid of the new norm of more data. It is, in fact, several times better than no data or patients mismanaging or misinterpreting their own data. Physicians will need to be prescriptive and tell patients how and when to use their devices. In my experience, patients rarely abuse the privilege of connectivity with their doctor. At least I know Doug, the federal agent, never did.

INTEGRATING SENSORS: CAN WE BRING IT ALL TOGETHER?

Real-time remote monitoring will be an essential part of these sensor strategies. Already, the large EMR datasets are challenging to manage with traditional software and commonly available data management tools. The moment we open this up to continuous streaming data, we have greatly increased the complexity. In health care, these data are overwhelming not only because of the volume but also because of the diversity in the data and the speed at which it is coming at us, creating the need for systems to handle this quickly and efficiently. These large datasets coming from sensor strategies only further the complexity of the problem of overwhelming data. Continuous and daily oversight of physiological parameters is central to managing chronic diseases and reducing readmissions and flare-ups. Operationalizing this will not be easy.

How does all this data streaming in on a continuous basis get assimilated into the workflow? It is complicated. We must objectively assess the added value of this information in caring for patients to justify the sensor and the collection of all this data. The clinical or business value here will come to fruition as these mHealth tools become a part of the workflow and payment models.

Integration of this into the EMR may or may not be a headache, depending on the approach taken. The federal government seems to be paying attention to the red tape and belabored process of this integration. They recently called for greater interoperability through an emerging data-exchange standard called Fast Healthcare Interoperability Resources (FHIR). The FHIR eases the impediments toward integration of third-party apps with the EMR. This allows for the digital tools to get directly merged with the EMR workflow, but not with the database. This always means that the mobile health data can be accessed through an embedded window within the EMR. But there is no need for opening a separate application to find this information. There is no need for any additional clicks.

As discussed earlier, the pandemic and the dawn of virtual care have already highlighted the rampant inequity in care and the large digital divide. The deployment of mHealth care may further this. Internet and smartphone adoption rates are lower in low-income, disabled, elderly, and rural populations. As innovative technology evolves and health care institutions begin creating and disseminating their own branded apps, it becomes imperative that a distinct effort be made to resource the disenfranchised and not unknowingly increase the disparities in care delivery.

The future does look quite good. It will become a lot more complex before it becomes exceedingly simple, and during that period we will continually second-guess our choices. Life, devices, and digital data will all converge. Nonetheless, it will remain our responsibility to ensure that these technological advances never undermine the human aspect of medicine.

PART II
VIRTUAL CARE

6

TELEHEALTH: FAD OR HERE TO STAY?

I am pretty sure people are going to start writing letters again once the email fad passes.
WILLIE GEIST

It was 8:55 a.m. and the ever-so-gentle "ting" on my laptop told me that Joan had just arrived in my virtual waiting room. All I had to do was click on the little green icon to let Joan into my home and allow me access to hers. Like Joan, I prefer not to use an artificial background and keep my backdrop real whether I am doing the virtual clinic from home or my hospital office, so it feels authentic and personal. There she was in her living room, beaming. Joan is an amazing, progressive eighty-seven-year-old who has spent much of her life traveling all over the world. The pandemic changed all this in an instant, and she was now holed up in her apartment in an assisted living facility. She had long-standing chronic obstructive lung disease and all the risk factors for falling severely ill from COVID. As a result, she had been confined to her living space, with not a single step outdoors for the last three months. So she was happy for any form of human contact.

We were both thrilled to see each other, and after exchanging pleasantries, she said, "Jag"—she has always called me by my first name—"I know you can't examine me over this tele-portal, but I have all my readings ready for you. My heart rate about thirty minutes ago was seventy-three; the upper blood pressure reading was one hundred and thirty and the lower one seventy. I do not have a fever, and my oxygen levels are ninety-three." She quickly added that she had invested in an oxygen saturation monitor because of the pandemic and her precarious lung situation. Pretty amazing! I jokingly asked her if she had listened to her own heart and lungs.

We talked about her A-fib and her heart disease for the next fifteen minutes. I was disturbed to hear that she'd had to completely stop taking daily walks because of the restrictions imposed within her living facility. It was tough to know whether she was symptomatic with exertion, as she was sedentary most of the time. There were no changes to make in her medications, and I began reassuring her and winding down my conversation. I had another patient to get to. Joan, however, would not let go. She wanted to chat. She pulled a photo frame from the center table and introduced me to her grandchildren, seven-year-old Martin and thirteen-year-old Ella. She was visibly upset that she could not hug them and spend time with them. I chatted with her for a few minutes, as I knew this was more than a consultation. It was her way of clutching a semblance of normalcy. Even though separated by large distances, we were close enough. I could tell from her animated speech and watching her breathing that she was fine. She was doing well, and her vital signs seemed to suggest the same.

Pre-pandemic, Joan was a habitual traveler and had developed many friendships across several countries. The pandemic forced her to learn how to keep in touch with her many acquaintances through her desktop computer. She also learned to record and measure her own vital signs so that she could provide objective information to help the clinician during the virtual clinical visit. She knew it was not safe for her to visit the hospital.

It took a pandemic for the inevitable to happen. The scathing viral infection kept everyone indoors, enforced masks and social distancing, and spurred the advent of virtual care, or what some refer to as telehealth. What had been in the works for more than a decade became a reality overnight. We were all forced to get on the virtual-care bandwagon through platforms such as Zoom, Facetime, Skype, and countless others. The chatter across Twitter and social media had initially been overwhelmingly positive. Virtual care became the backbone of the digital infrastructure that allowed patients and physicians to connect with each other. Remote visits and simple devices to monitor vital signs and weight began the advent of a novel patient experience. This was the start of supervised care from a distance, a changing patient-provider relationship, and evolving expectations in how patients wanted to receive their care.

THE UPTICK!

We went from zero to sixty in milliseconds. Even prior to 2019, digital strategies had begun to bubble up, and then the pandemic came and added high-octane jet fuel to the simmer. Tele-visits began to Zoom beyond belief. Microsoft, Zoom, Teladoc, Amwell, and other videoconferencing companies began to have a field day. Along with their usage, their stocks skyrocketed. In less than a year of the pandemic, more than four hundred million tele-visits had occurred in the United States alone, with an expanding business proposition for telehealth valued at nearly $200 billion by 2026.

Going back to the period prior to the pandemic, fewer than 10 percent of patients surveyed were interested in virtual care. Most patients and physicians preferred personal contact, and the insurers themselves were reluctant to pay, as they felt that tele-visits could be a slippery slope and result in excessive use. As COVID-19 afflicted millions across the world, it gave new life to this mode of medicine. The intent was twofold: the ability to treat the rising number of COVID patients in the hospital while safeguarding the well-being of our vulnerable non-COVID patients by keeping them at home. Beyond this, it also reduced the need for personal protective equipment, which was in short supply and indispensable for the protection of frontline health care workers. Virtual care was here to provide easy access to clinicians while enabling social distancing.

By the end of 2020, more than a billion patients had access to telehealth across the globe. Earlier that year, at the World Medical Innovation Forum 2020 in Boston, in a survey of fifty health care CEOs, more than 85 percent agreed that patients would continue to travel less (post-pandemic), and 100 percent of them felt that the use of telemedicine would increase significantly to cater to this change. In a separate survey of patients at the same time, nearly 60 percent of respondents stated they were more likely to continue to use telehealth services, and more than one-third would even change their providers to ones who offered tele-visits. That this was more than a trend became obvious when a quarter said they would prefer virtual care, even if they had to self-pay without insurance coverage. What's interesting was that despite most leadership circles across the world knowing several years in advance that the rise in telehealth was inevitable, it took a global catastrophe, a true black-swan event, to accelerate its overnight acceptance and adoption.

LOVE IT OR HATE IT—IT'S HERE TO STAY

Telemedicine, like everything else in medicine, abides by the one-third rule. One-third of patients hate it, one-third love it, and one-third are indifferent. Approximately one-third of physicians across all age-groups have an innate aversion to the potential virtues of virtual care. They would rather preserve their trade the way they initially learned to practice it. Much of that stems from the many years of in-person visits and the value and comfort perceived in social interaction with their patients. Some of this is also generational.

Among patients, as expected, the millennials and Gens X and Z comprise the largest cohort of supporters for this new way of life. But the boomers are not too far behind. Most grandparents, octa- and nonagenarians such as Joan, have learned to Zoom, Skype, Facetime, and use a variety of virtual tools. And, in fact, patients are now unwilling and hesitant to come into hospitals and wait in crowded waiting areas. There is this overarching fear of breathing in the exhaled air of a stranger. Who knows what the guy on the seat next to you may be expelling with each breath? It seems very plausible that this hesitancy will convert to a habit and then become the norm for a wide swath of vulnerable patients with comorbidities who don't feel safe coming to hospitals and may be at high risk of becoming a target for a communicable disease. So how will the current infrastructure of care evolve? There is no simple answer, but it is something we will discuss at greater length in the last section of the book, which examines "sustainable disruptions."

The funding for digital health at the beginning of 2020 was looking pretty good to start. There was already venture capital flowing into this arena. A lot of money (more than $300 billion invested) flowed in during the first quarter of 2020, and the pandemic further fueled its escalation. Evidently, telemedicine is becoming the playing field of larger health care and digital companies alongside a horde of start-ups that are racing to fill the needs of the larger rigid hospital systems and academic medical centers. Several of the larger health care companies, including Philips Healthcare, GE Healthcare, Cerner Corporation, IBM, McKesson, AMD Global Telemedicine, Amwell, and Honeywell Life Care Solutions, have already made inroads. They are putting into place constructs to make the patient experience top-notch. They are in the midst of creating individualized digital platforms that can wrap their arms around patients through the course of their entire out- and inpatient clinical life cycle. This is complicated and has not been without a struggle.

It does seem perplexing that even though digital strategies have invaded all forms of daily living, such as ordering candles, diapers, or yoga pants on Amazon; hailing cars; booking travel; dining; or banking, the one place that has continued to stay siloed is the health care industry. Probably, it is the complexity of the many in-person interactions and multiple other touch points, including imaging, laboratory tests, procedures, and so on, that have contributed to the slow takeover. Telehealth, with its virtual interactive framework, provides the humanistic appeal to the expanding footprint of digital health. Besides enhancing access, efficiency, patient experience, and potentially clinical outcomes, cost savings seem to be a big draw. Goldman Sachs estimates that digitizing several aspects of health care could result in savings exceeding hundreds of billions of dollars. More than two-thirds of these savings will come from management of chronic diseases. The bigger question revolves around how these digital health companies fit into the world two to ten years from now and what they will fulfill in the long term.

Care delivery must be about accepting the need to meet patients where they are and when they need care. To that end, the pandemic and the quick adoption of telehealth epitomizes that it may be useful to be the disruptor rather than to be disrupted. Sometimes, even though the macro economy within the health care arena may indicate that it is going to be difficult to raise capital to pursue digital strategies, it may just be the right time to pivot. Boris Groysberg, a professor from the Harvard Business School, has nicely stated that in times like this, it is important to protect your core strengths and pivot to new opportunities to grow. It is our time now to be ready to pivot to providing care at a distance, with telehealth and digital care seeming the most apt way to fill that need. It is important to recognize that this will not replace the in-person visit but will serve as a useful adjunct or a complementary mode of care. If we truly want to increase access and equitable care while scaling the capacity of giving instantaneous care, then telehealth is going to remain a part of our arsenal. It is here to stay.

STUFF GETS MISSED

I think it's safe to say that anyone who has seen a doctor in the past few months has been offered the possibility of a virtual visit. Folks are overjoyed at not having to travel, drive, park, wait, and navigate the complexity of the hospital, and thereby sacrifice a large part of their day. But then, it's important to recognize that a tele-visit is not a one-size-fits-all strategy. It is but an entry point, a foyer into a multidimensional, ever-evolving building complex, with unique experiences adapted to each individual's needs.

As a practicing cardiologist, I have always been a strong proponent for telehealth; however, I have to profess that medical care is complicated and there are many conditions that require an in-person clinical exam and laboratory tests. Otherwise, stuff gets missed . . . to a much larger extent than during an in-person visit. Every now and again there are some unfortunate tales to recount. Quite recently a patient of mine, who despite appearing stable over a video consultation, had to be admitted the very next day with severe heart failure. The swelling of the legs and the distension of neck veins (signs of heart failure) could not be easily seen over the video. This is not uncommon. This is where virtual care serves as an adjunct and not a replacement to in-person care. It may not come as a surprise to most, but there will always be considerable value to the clinical examination. Moreover, most clinicians can do with some additional training in asking more trenchant questions and adopting modified clinical examinations to avoid missing stuff.

Similarly, a colleague's patient recently developed critical limb ischemia and early gangrene of the right foot. This was despite frequent virtual visits, where the incipient and slow progression of reduced blood supply to the leg and foot was missed because of the absence of an in-person clinical exam—it is tough to see the leg well over a webcam. Notably, the patient was also underplaying his symptoms since he did not want to have to come to the hospital, due to his fear of catching COVID. The situation got bad enough that his right foot had to be amputated.

Patients with kidney or liver disease really need laboratory tests and a clinical exam to ascertain the stability or progression of their clinical condition. Virtual visits in isolation do not cut it. However, combining those telehealth appointments with point-of-care testing (using apps) or laboratory tests performed closer to home makes the clinical assessment a more robust one. The other day, my patient kept coughing during a virtual consultation, and I had to urgently orchestrate an in-person visit because I really needed to put my stethoscope on the patient's chest to hear the breath sounds and assess the level of congestion or rule out pneumonia. There is often a need for some quantitative laboratory testing or a chest X-ray (as in this case) to back up a clinical hunch.

We often take for granted the importance of nonverbal cues that are picked up in an in-person visit. During virtual visits, looking directly at the patient's face for the duration of the visit, one can miss the fidgeting of the hands, or the nervous tic that the patient may be trying to suppress. Even eye contact can sometimes prove challenging as a result of the location of their web camera or the angle of their laptop or phone. Perhaps most importantly, expressing empathy or providing comfort across a camera is not particularly easy; sometimes just a touch of the hand is so much more meaningful than anything we can tell our patients. However, there is something to be said for the connection established outside the concrete walls of a hospital environment.

Many of us reminisce about the era of medical house calls with nostalgia. Now we can relive it. And we can do so in a twenty-first-century, tech-savvy way. In addition to increased access, efficiency, and positive patient experience, tele-visits allow us a glimpse into each other's lives. Personally, it has often strengthened a preexisting relationship I may have had with a patient who otherwise I have always seen in an in-office environment. I get to meet Grandma, see the baby, and even get a glimpse of the four-legged friend. It has given me an opportunity to effectively teach the patient to care for themselves in their home environment—something that we try to do abstractly in the outpatient clinic.

Tele-visits are not for everybody and certainly not for every clinical condition. A shared-decision approach (between the patient and the doctor) helps crystallize which visits should be virtual versus should be in person. We have seen telehealth usage mirror each of the surges during the pandemic. Every viral variant peak was associated with a concomitant increase in the use of virtual visits, as patients were inclined to avoid venturing out of their homes. Despite the recurrent need for telehealth, there remains the fear that regulatory barriers eased during the height of the pandemic will be reversed and reimbursement for services provided will be scaled back. This will cause the telehealth pendulum to swing back, closer to where it was in the pre-pandemic era. There are already edicts coming down the line that out-of-state consultation via telehealth is not allowed. The patient needs to be within the state border to legally have a consultation, even if they have been seen in the past by the same clinician for an in-person consultation. As crazy as this may sound, some desperate patients from adjoining states are driving just beyond the state border and then engaging in their virtual consultation using their smartphone from their car. It will be a while before states break down barriers to allow for a national license for practicing clinical medicine, but the idea of interstate reciprocity has been suggested and may come to fruition.

The long-term trends will be dictated by the consumer. Patients and their expectations will drive the change where it needs to be. Also, as we develop new sensor strategies that can digitize each organ of the body and remotely provide more quantitative and actionable data that can replace the conventional clinical exam, telehealth will get even more traction.

REPLACING THE CONVENTIONAL CLINICAL EXAM

The physical exam with the in-person consultation has been the cornerstone of the patient-doctor encounter for centuries, since the detection of disease. The recognition of master clinicians was tied to their ability in eliciting clinical signs and making a correct diagnosis. In the past, most illnesses were essentially diagnosed through touching the patient. This could involve holding the wrist to feel the pulse, the subtleties of which go beyond just a simple measure of heart rate. Any change in regularity, volume, or upstroke of the pulse can help diagnose a spectrum of cardiac and noncardiac diseases. The physical exam involves a visual inspection of the hair, eyes, head, and neck while palpating and feeling for swellings. This also includes a careful examination of the neck for the pulsating pattern of the carotids and the rhythmic undulations of the jugular veins. And then a methodical examination of the chest, abdomen, and the extremities, all in one systematic swoop from head to toe. Besides the tactile and sensory feedback from the individual organs during the clinical exam, it also involved placing one's ear on the chest or back to listen to the lungs and heart until the advent of the listening tube, or what later came to be recognized as the stethoscope. The stethoscope became an essential part of the repertoire and served to legitimize the clinician and the role. The orderly inspection, palpation, percussion, and auscultation of the human body provided clues to its internal disease states. This examination usually occurs in an examination room, with a directed conversation aimed at unraveling the cause of the illness. The patient-doctor encounter is a sensory experience on both sides—one that involves touch, sound, sight, and smell. When asked, patients have always stated that they appreciate the hands-on examination. This is more for the affective component rather than the expected accuracy of the evaluation. Touch has always been central to this encounter and demonstrates concern, empathy, warmth, and the humanness of the caregiver.

In recent years, though, the stethoscope has begun to acquire an ornamental status, and before long may become a relic. There is an ongoing effort to deconstruct the human body into an assembly of organs, the functionality of each then being picked up by sensors and transmitted as continuous digital data in time and space. This would enable a virtual exam that could potentially be more objective and unbiased but could be handicapped by the absence of human contact. Maybe that is acceptable, if the result is better or comparable to the in-person visit. The tele-visit needs to be a simple single portal that allows its integration with a suite of digital tools inclusive of texting, sensors, apps, and AI. It needs a multidongle, or a Swiss Army knife–equivalent plug-in of multiple diagnostic tools to facilitate the medical exam. These could include a remote handheld ultrasound, a digital stethoscope, and apps and wearables to measure temperature, heart rate, blood pressure, oxygen saturations, and other relevant clinical parameters. And beyond this, advanced computing, 3D holographic visualizations, and the science of haptics may, in the coming years, be a surrogate for the entire experience. This fits in with the pervasive non-touch culture taking over our everyday life and living. Possibly, some patients may become averse to a physician laying their bare or even gloved hands on them.

THE NON-TOUCH CULTURE

The mandate for masks and social distancing has helped further this rising contact-free culture. The slow herd immunity (with mutant strains) and fear of other contagions have already affected our behavior and begun to further entrench many of the pandemic-induced practice patterns. Greater automation (e.g., online banking and shopping) had been on the rise even prior to the pandemic and continues to increase. The McKinsey Global Institute has estimated that 60 percent of all jobs could see greater than 30 percent of key elements automated, potentially affecting more than five hundred million jobs globally.

The same is happening in the hospital environment. Human contact, hugs, high fives, and handshakes have become rare. Even prior to the pandemic, a greater reliance on testing and imaging had already made the physical exam redundant, at least to some extent. Not only do outpatient tele-visits preclude a physical exam, but somehow that culture has begun to find its way into the inpatient environment. Morning rounds at many hospitals have already become remote. The residents, consultants, and nurses huddle together in a conference room and tele-visit each patient's room. In-person visits are often door-side rather than bedside. It's a slippery slope, and the descent seems to have already begun.

Perhaps in certain inpatient situations, the physical exam may not add enough value. I remember my personal experience as a COVID patient, where the attending physician usually came in with a resident, neither of whom really examined me. But then again, in that situation, there was not a whole lot to gather from the in-person exam. Much of the evaluation of my clinical status was centered on my temperature, heart rate, blood pressure, and oxygen saturations, which could be easily acquired from the monitor, a thermometer, and a simple finger sensor. It did not make sense for the clinicians looking after me to be unnecessarily exposed to the virus. Sometimes the rounds were not bedside, not even door-side, but a video visit from outside the closed door to my room. Did this suitably replace the few minutes of in-person interaction? I will say no. The remote evaluation sometimes makes the patient wonder whether anybody truly cares.

It was during this period that I realized that every opportunity for in-person conversation was a privilege. I promised myself to work at it and practice it. Having said that, non-touch culture is here. As it becomes more pervasive, expectations will change, and a few years down the line, the next generation will consider much of this to be the norm. Some of us may long for the good old days, but then a fading memory will be transcribed over by a swift, efficient, more personalized, yet impersonal system. Maybe it will be "tone over touch" and AI-assisted interpretation of verbal and nonverbal cues. Let's make sure we continue to find ways of keeping it human and personal and always retain touch in our repertoire.

Telemedicine is transformative in that it changes these sensory dimensions of practice and the social encounter. We know that the in-person visit involves a much more personalized sensory experience and is comprised of touch, hearing, smell, and vision. The tele-visit does not provide this and involves the use of digital stethoscopes, thermometers, weighing scales, heart rate and blood pressure monitors, and oxygen saturation monitors with high-definition cameras on laptops, desktops, or in health kiosks. These health kiosks are being rolled out in workplaces, pharmacies, and supermarkets. A health checkup on the go, without disrupting a normal workday.

It is not clear whether virtual touch will ever equate to that of an in-person one. With advancing technology, will the sensory perception via the digital device be comparable to an in-person visit? Will the objectivity of the digital data be superior to the qualitative physical exam? But there are other places that virtual care has become a godsend, especially when more than one caregiver is involved in the decision-making process of a complex clinical situation that needs input from more than one specialty.

Clinical practice has evolved to where we always put the patient at the center and construct the care pathway around the patient, as opposed to the patient trying to figure out the care strategy. The practice of medicine is swiftly changing with a recognition of multidisciplinary care as the cornerstone. The big question that comes to mind is how telehealth will adapt to multidisciplinary care. For example, a patient with cancer often must meet with the oncologist, the radiation therapy specialist, the surgeon, and the imaging specialist, among sometimes a host of other supporting specialties. This is complicated enough as is, in terms of coordinating schedules and visits. Meetings are staggered, and specialists get pulled away from other tasks they may have. Multidisciplinary care requires a team approach and communication to enable the formalizing of an individualized treatment approach. These can be complicated meetings, and if there are family members in attendance, the clinic rooms can be congested and overbearing. This is where telehealth provides a significant edge, especially when the encounter is primarily cognitive. Everyone joins through a video visit, screens are shared, imaging and laboratory results are pulled up and discussed in a transparent way with the patient and family members, and a collective treatment approach is settled upon.

We have already begun doing this routinely for our patients with heart failure and implanted devices. We have the cardiac electrophysiologist, the heart failure specialist, the imaging doctor, and patient's cardiologist, along with the patient and the family as needed, all show up face-to-face through the video-visit format. This can be done more flexibly from remote locations, accommodating everyone's commitments and schedules. Not to mention the avoided stress for the patient not having to come to the hospital and deal with transportation, parking, and so forth. We share information about the echocardiographic images of the heart, the streams of data emanating from the implanted devices, along with a discussion of the patient's medications and current clinical condition, then collectively come together to make a plan. This may involve adjusting medications, further education on lifestyle adaptations, or programming of the device in a more individualized manner. And if any of this involves or needs an in-person visit, it gets set up at that time. This system works well, and informal surveys have demonstrated very high patient satisfaction.

Dr. Rasmussen, chief clinical officer and neurosurgeon at Cleveland Clinic, has posted on social media that he only sees patients virtually, especially in the context of a complex neurosurgical practice. He states, "All I need to do is talk to you and see your imaging." He is of the belief (as are many other like-minded clinicians) that mandating in-person visits is archaic and quaint. In line with this, the concept of "virtual first" primary care visits is also speedily gaining traction.

TRADITIONALIST VS. VIRTUALIST

Having practiced medicine for more than a couple of decades, I could be considered a traditionalist. That may not be too far from the truth, as I have always enjoyed seeing my patients in person. I like the handshakes and love the hugs. I enjoy the one-on-one, face-to-face encounters and most of all cherish the long-term personal relationships I have with most of my patients. Beyond all the textbook knowledge, I depend on my instincts and my visual in-person evaluation and physical exam of the patient to bolster my clinical assessment and recommendations. On the flip side, I also enjoy the virtual experience. It allows me to be a guest in the homes or offices of my patients and gives me a different vantage point. The tone of the visit is quite different from the one in the hospital clinic. My primary purpose as a physician is to make my patient feel well, and also alleviate their anxiety around their heart problems. If making them happy and less anxious means seeing them virtually and not in an intimidating hospital environment, then so be it. But it does on many occasions handicap my ability to evaluate my patient three-dimensionally, hold their hand, feel their wrist, or listen to their heart. The risk of missing something clinically significant (like impending gangrene, as described earlier) in the absence of an objective exam and nonverbal cues often makes me second-guess myself.

Nevertheless, I am prepared to meet the patient wherever she or he may desire, in the clinic or virtual office. The traditionalist must accept that the clinic appointment is not about them, but about the patient. It is about finding the right type of visit to make it convenient, comfortable, and most apt for a patient, depending on the underlying disease state. No "virtualist" can be good enough without having a sound foundation in and understanding of the traditional practice of in-person medicine. And in the current era, restricting oneself to just the traditionalist approach means not adapting to the changing times. It is possible to blend caring and compassion with convenience and meeting your patients where they want to be met. The future state is a hybrid one, and the proportion of traditional versus virtual care will depend on the type of medicine one practices. For example, a cardiologist, a pulmonologist, a primary care physician, or an orthopedic surgeon will all have a different blend of this fusion. It is not about the traditionalist versus the virtualist anymore. It is about understanding the patient and their illness and determining the right way to see them in the right place. Experience will teach us which patients with which illness may best be seen virtually versus traditionally and how often. There is concern that opening the floodgates on telehealth may result in excessive and unnecessary care, rendering health care even more expensive. Many questions remain to be answered: What is the right mix? Is it really the right way forward? Can we afford this, and is it sustainable? These issues and the sustainability of telehealth are discussed in greater detail in the next chapter.

NEXT STEP—THE METAVERSE?

Telehealth will evolve beyond video visits into the world of the metaverse, which constitutes a form of parallel reality. It is a shared virtual three-dimensional space accessed over the internet that brings the digital and physical worlds together. It allows for an immersive, interactive experience by individuals separated by large distances across the globe. This metaverse allows for virtual but real-enough experiences that give a feeling of being there. All it needs is a headset that can incorporate virtual reality, augmented reality, and mixed reality aided by artificial intelligence. The metaverse of medicine can provide a realistic patient-doctor experience in a virtual clinic room. Add to this sensor-derived data, and you have an in-person equivalent visit, even when physically apart. Of course, this comes with its own challenges, of privacy, interoperability, regulations, and licensures to practice across geographic boundaries and in the metaverse.

Despite these barriers, entrepreneurs have begun dipping their toes into this ocean. Clinical initiatives have already started, especially in the mental health world. The metaverse may be the ideal way of treating situational phobias (e.g., of airplanes, heights, or closed spaces), PTSD, anxiety, and hallucinations. The virtual world allows the psychologist or psychiatrist to recreate the clinical situation while providing a supportive environment during the event. Also, post-surgery rehabilitation will transcend from virtual video visits to the metaverse arena, where personal exercise guidance can be provided. Post-COVID, with more than 95 percent of health care facilities having the ability to provide telehealth visits, the metaverse seems the natural next step.

7

ARE WE BREAKING THE BANK?

Too much of anything is the beginning of a mess.
DOROTHY DRAPER

It was my fourth virtual visit for the morning. I was on a roll. It was just perfect. Without stepping away from my desk, I had finished three virtual visits, and by the end of each, I had even completed my clinic notes. It doesn't get better than that. I love seeing my patients, but categorically, like most physicians, I hate writing clinic notes to encapsulate the entire clinic visit. I frequently get reminders from the administrators that my clinic notes are incomplete and cannot be submitted for billing. That bothers me even more since I am already working pretty hard.

Routinely, one can finish a thirty-minute visit and then spend another thirty minutes trying to finish completing the notes that succinctly span the breadth and depth of the conversation, list out the clinical problems, and detail a potential plan for each of them. It's important to be thorough about these; otherwise the next time you see the patient, you may have no idea what you recommended in the prior visit. This is especially challenging if you have hundreds of patients on your panel, a failing memory, or limited typing skills to keep up. All of which seem to be problems I have.

Telehealth visits have made that easy, as you are looking into the camera of your computer, and many times you can type away at your keyboard while still maintaining eye contact. There is no running to the waiting room to greet your patient and then to the clinic room to see them. The moment you switch on the camera and let them in from your virtual waiting room, there is dedicated one-on-one time with the patient. But then not everything goes smoothly. Technical issues are always waiting to mess up your day and throw you off schedule. And today, just like on most clinic days, there was another technical problem serving to distract and annoy.

I was waiting to let Beth, a sixty-three-year-old real estate agent and a patient of mine for more than a decade, into my virtual clinic. She was checked in for a Zoom appointment, and I was already into my tenth minute of waiting to let her in. By the indicators on my computer screen, I could tell that she had logged in for the video visit but was unable to cross the final hurdle to get into my virtual waiting room. I knew for sure that she was computer savvy and that there was obviously some glitch. I waited a little longer and now was fifteen minutes into her scheduled visit time. I was seeing her after a year and knew I needed to spend time with her; the clock was ticking, and I was going to be thrown off schedule by thirty minutes. That would be a disaster, especially because of the downstream spiraling effect on all my subsequent patients. So I picked up the phone to call her after getting her phone number from the electronic medical record. I found her landline busy, so I tried her cell. She picked up and was on the other line with the technical help section from my hospital. I could hear frustration in her voice as she repeated words such as *the blue icon*, *double click*, and *pop-up blocker*. Clearly, she was having a bad day. I asked her to get off the call with technical support and decided to expedite the visit over the phone. I would have FaceTimed her, but I knew that was not a cybersecure strategy and could violate HIPAA rules. We chatted for the next twenty minutes and set a follow-up in-person visit for a year later. Three patient visits later the same afternoon, the same problem occurred with another patient. It was not a good day.

MONEY = CHANGE

Telehealth is no panacea. It is not without its problems. The presence of technical issues and the lack of objective evaluations to complement clinic visits will continue to haunt its implementation. Beyond this, the wavering policies regarding impending regulatory and reimbursement changes will remain a looming threat. Although a robust telehealth program may be a necessary tool for the future, it may not be allowed to realize its fullest potential. Because of these uncertainties and the potentially waning COVID era, the barriers for in-person visits will also drop, and it may not be too long before we revert to our old ways. When the first COVID surge looked to be getting under control, the medical community observed signs of a quick rewind in practice patterns. Telemedicine use plummeted as early as three months post the start of the COVD season in the US, and by the end of 2020 had dropped to a threateningly pre-pandemic level. And then came the delta, followed by the omicron surge, and patients again did not want to come. As a result, there was that all-too-familiar uptick. But why this reticence, this urge to drift away from remote medicine and fall back into our old ways?

First, putting telemedicine into play is resource intensive, and a physician practice needs not only to invest in the appropriate technology but also to train staff and patients to use it. It is particularly challenging to have enough staff to teach and train the elderly or individual patients who are not familiar with the technology, especially when it comes to participating in a video visit. Notably, these video visits require new workflows, schedules, documentation protocols, and so on. Larger institutions and organizations with the appropriate resources and expertise have been able to shift into the telehealth lanes with secure platforms, while smaller organizations have found it problematic. Coordinating laboratory testing and imaging at a remote site has its own challenges. A few of these hurdles have resulted in the inertia seen within some practices or may be the cause for the quick reversion to the way things used be. Also, there needs to be more to it than just offering the service. It is about enhancing the experience, creating the rapport, providing the support, and building the trust. A single bad digital experience can be off-putting and could be the death knell for the adoption of telehealth for some patients.

During the pandemic, care transcended borders and boundaries. It was okay to be looking after patients across state borders. The need to have a prior relationship with their clinician was not absolutely necessary. Patients and providers could be seeing each other for the first time in a virtual consultation. Also, the use of less-regulated platforms and waivers to make telehealth more flexible with the use of telephone calls were in play. But not for long. In mid-2021, the emergency mandates around telehealth were reversed. There was a rollback on practicing across state lines and looming variability in parity of reimbursement for in-person versus tele-visits across different states. The pendulum had swung back. The lack of permanence to the reimbursement structure and the continuing variability in payments within state Medicaid or private health plans intensified the reluctance. Many of the large private insurers that had held back on the need for copayments for a telehealth visit were raring to slap on these prerequisites again. The direction and amount of money flow determine the extent and the shape of the change. Money dictates practice culture . . . and change.

EASY ACCESS = MORE CARE

Will easy access lead to more care and greater expense? Some of this may already be happening; previously no-charge-rendered patient-doctor telephone calls are now being converted into reimbursable telephone virtual visits. There is also something to be said about multiple ineffective tele-visits to monitor a condition that may require a single in-person exam to provide more meaningful care. Maybe some of this could be corrected by the future availability of sensor technology to provide objective and unbiased assessments of the clinical situation. As sensor approaches are offered, many of the negative attributes we see about missing clinical indicators of severity will diminish over time. Currently, as a result of this lack of objective assessment, different specialties are embracing telehealth with varying levels of enthusiasm.

Dermatology has made some big inroads with telehealth, for example. A large part of dermatology is a spot diagnosis looking at a skin lesion. Whether it is acne, psoriasis, eczema, or dermatitis, these can be assessed quite easily via a video visit. The acne patient's response to medications such as isotretinoin does not need an in-person visit. Many AI algorithms being currently studied could help the nonspecialist make a diagnosis of a skin disorder from a picture. One can only be certain that, as technology evolves, patients at some point in time may have access to these algorithms to make a self-diagnosis before even consulting the doctor. How this all plays out will be determined by the accuracy of the algorithm, the risk of over- and under-diagnosis, and the downstream impact on the use of resources.

The pandemic has exposed our vulnerabilities as individuals and as a society. There has been a significant uptick in the utilization of telehealth for behavioral problems such as anxiety, domestic violence, and depression. Most of these demands are a direct reflection of the impact of COVID on our societal structure and interactions. Telehealth in this arena has been a boon, as it not only provides access but also enhances privacy and helps some patients to have an open conversation. It is less inhibiting and intimidating than an in-person, face-to-face conversation. Besides patients, many health care and frontline workers have availed themselves of these services during the COVID period.

Even rheumatology, a specialty that significantly relies on the physical exam to make a diagnosis, shifted course. It was always thought to be challenging to distinguish joint tenderness due to bone or muscular pain from a swelling due to an inflammatory process without a physical exam. Despite this, tele-rheumatology gained significant traction during the pandemic. To ease the concerns of some of the naysayers, the American College of Rheumatology published a statement on tele-rheumatology suggesting that there remains a reasonable role for virtual visits in this space. They emphasized "the role of telemedicine as a tool with the potential to increase access and improve care for patients with rheumatic diseases, but it should not replace essential face-to-face assessments at medically appropriate intervals." Clinicians often ask their patients to do maneuvers to assist with the diagnosis, or send pictures or show their rash over the video visit to assist in making the diagnosis and helping gauge the clinical severity of the disease. The management of joint diseases relies greatly on ancillary services such as imaging, joint injections, and the administration of biologic infusions. Even though these are critical to the economics of the practice of rheumatology, telehealth-aided administration of home IV therapies with remote monitoring for safety is finding its way into care delivery.

Another form of digital care transformation has been a remote algorithm-driven disease management platform. One such program at Mass General Brigham in Boston uses pharmacists and health care navigators, supported by a specialist, to look after a large populace of patients. The objective is to help patients manage their cholesterol and blood pressure in a personalized way with target goals. Similar to Joan, our eighty-seven-year-old, most patients have begun seeking objectivity from their telehealth visits. They have started to familiarize themselves with taking their vital signs in preparation for their clinical encounter. Over-the-counter blood pressure monitors, heart rate and rhythm monitoring devices, oxygen saturation sensors, and thermometers, along with a slew of wellness apps, have begun to find their way into many primary care, cardiac, and pulmonary virtual visits. App-based cognitive behavioral therapy has also begun to get more traction in treating depression and body dysmorphic disorders and has shown to improve the quality of life. The previously paternalistic practice of medicine is being transformed to one that is patient-centric and promotes patient empowerment and partnership.

CREEP AND CARE EVERYWHERE

Before the pandemic, telehealth delivery was incredibly varied and not well centralized. Much of it was localized within a single service line (for example, tele-neurology, providing stroke services, tele-ICU, tele-counseling) or just a few providers using the technology when they could for a particular fixed-use case. Tele-neurology is one of these, providing emergent care to stroke patients in community hospitals that lack cutting-edge interventional strategies of care. But now the role has expanded, the adoption has been propelled forth and so have the indications. In medicine there is a well-accepted concept known as "indication creep." This means that an accepted treatment strategy for a particular group of patients with an illness may expand to a subset that was not previously tested or indicated for that treatment strategy. As an example, there are some treatments that have been specifically studied and tested in very severe rheumatoid arthritis, late stages of cancer, or fulminant lung infections, and shown to be of significant benefit. Using this as a justification, it is not unusual for physicians to push the envelope and try the same treatment in patients with milder forms of those disease states, even if that therapeutic modality has not been evaluated in that subset of patients. We might see this in telehealth across several use cases, as doctors begin pushing the boundaries on what can and cannot be seen virtually, especially as the comfort level grows with accompanying disease-specific sensor modalities, transmitting impartial information of the clinical state.

Another form of creep that will occur is a "border creep." The global adoption of telehealth and accessibility of clinicians across state and national borders will change the playing field of how patients will seek care. The forward-thinking institutions that begin to make the leap here to becoming global caregivers will find that, in a few years, they will have diverse portfolios that will make them more sustainable. Even though at this stage, the regulatory barriers and state-centric approaches within the US may serve as deterrents, this will over time be the natural progression of the delivery of health care.

When we talk about telehealth, the competition is not local or within one's community. It is not competition from the local CVS or Walmart. It is more about what is going to happen on the national and global landscape. If you want to see a dermatologist, you could see one at the opposite end of the country or even seek consultation from a dermatologist from the premier institutes in Germany or the UK, or anywhere else in the world. Strategies to leverage consultative services will be real-time and authenticated through regulatory bodies in the future. The fifth generation (5G) of wireless technology is already here, enhancing the speed of this discourse. And the 6G network is going to further lead to this aspect of care exploding. The sixth generation of wireless technology can deliver peak data rates of eight thousand gigabits per second with a delay of less than one hundred microseconds. This is a hundred times faster than 5G. It will be a game changer. The bandwidth and the ability to send large files with low latency will enable faster decisions and, in some cases, allow for international multidisciplinary teams coming together virtually in real time to help make decisions. Despite the potential regulatory barriers, red tape, and restrictions, much of this change will be driven by the expectations of the consumer—the patient. The transition from creep to crawl to soar is in the making.

OVER-CARE COULD BREAK THE BANK

When addressing the financial implications of this technology, it becomes important to separate out what this is in the COVID era versus what it could be in the post-COVID era. In the early weeks of COVID, most institutions and practices were not seeing patients, and consequently were depleting their cash on hand. There was essentially no outpatient office or in-hospital activity besides that comprising primarily COVID patients. The revenue of practices would have dried up had it not been for telehealth coming in to save patients and practices. At most institutions, including Massachusetts General Hospital, more than 80 percent of visits across all specialties and primary care had switched quickly to telemedicine. At times this was as high as nearly 100 percent, all in a matter of weeks. The federal government soon came to the rescue, providing pay parity for virtual care and in-person visits.

There are two long-term positive fiscal impacts on the overall health care expenditure. These include a lower price per virtual visit compared to an in-person visit, coupled with the savings from reduced diagnostic testing. Recently, an interesting study compared the extent of utilization of services accompanying tele-visits versus in-person visits during nonurgent care. Tele-visits resulted in fewer lab tests and X-rays compared to an in-person check at a retail health clinic, urgent care center, or primary care physician. Notably, a telehealth visit was nearly $200 cheaper than a visit to the PCP's office or $2,000 less compared to an ER visit.

There also are well-established telehealth-facilitated subspecialty programs (e.g., telestroke) that provide rural and less-privileged environments access to specialty care otherwise not available. Strokes are infrequent, complicated, high-stakes events that require immediate care and expertise that is not available in half the ERs across the country. The telestroke programs of tertiary hospitals provide the opportunity for immediate interventions to reestablish blood flow that can significantly improve outcome and reduce disability. Intermountain Healthcare's telehealth program showed that it reduced the chances of a newborn from the neonatal intensive care unit needing to be transferred to a larger hospital by almost 30 percent. That amounted to roughly sixty-seven fewer transfers in a year, and a savings of $1,220,352 for the health system. There remains variability still on the return on investment and extent of reimbursement. Even though many payers are currently reimbursing tele-visits at in-person visit rates, this may not remain the case in the future. It's all in a state of flux.

The best reimbursement rate for telehealth remains to be determined. Multiple factors will influence this. Will this morph into every transaction having a fee for service, or will this be a capitated strategy leaving it to the physicians to decide how many visits they truly need to ensure good outcomes, but under the umbrella of a fixed payment per patient? (I will discuss this in greater detail in Part IV, Chapters 17 and 18.) There is the fear that the ease and convenience of telehealth will result in increased utilization and, in turn, spending. There is also some angst that care provided without objective evaluations and tests may result in poor decisions and suboptimal treatment plans prescribed by the clinician. This could in turn affect outcomes and have a negative impact on costs to the system. There is evidence now that telehealth can reduce the need for urgent care and ER visits. Also, based on the savings described above, one can clearly see that for some chronic-condition exacerbations, several tele-visits may serve a patient more than a single ER visit. The hope is that timely tele-visits will prevent the worsening of a clinical condition, thereby preventing hospitalization. We can't afford to let this break the bank; patients and the doctors both need to understand their role and make it sustainable.

CHRONIC DISEASE CARE = SAVINGS

Matt McGregor is a sixty-three-year-old retired math teacher who has diabetes, hypertension, and chronic obstructive lung disease. He has had a heart attack in the past and also suffers from end-stage renal disease, besides being treated for prostate cancer with hormonal therapy. This is not at all unusual. Most patients, as they get older, develop multiple chronic diseases, each independently influencing outcome and collectively compounding the negative influence on the patient's health. Lifestyle, sleep patterns, behavioral health, nutrition, and exercise are of paramount importance in their impact on the clinical outcome of the patient. Knowing that I would have problems with Matt getting engaged in his own care and choices, I enrolled him in the video group visit program for diabetes and hypertension. It was here that he was able to connect with a digital community of other patients living his exact same life. He could finally commiserate and simultaneously get inspired by his digital community.

Undoubtedly, chronic disease is one of the biggest drivers of health care spending. Six of every ten patients have chronic disease, and four of ten may have two chronic conditions. Three of every four dollars spent on health care in the United States are spent on chronic diseases. And the CDC has reported that diabetes, heart disease, and cancer (all three of which Matt McGregor has) are the most common chronic diseases causing death, and the leading drivers of the United States' $3.58 trillion in annual health care costs. The change in our demographic profile, with an aging population, has further added to this fiscal burden. The conventional practice of scheduled twenty- to thirty-minute visits on a quarterly basis is not enough to provide care that accounts for the complexity of different conditions and their interactions. Clearly quarterly visits are not enough to prevent flare-ups and are unmistakably suboptimal in preventing readmissions. It is here that virtual care coupled with digital monitoring (as previously described) and home-based interventions will change the care paradigm. But is this care pathway reserved for the privileged? We know that patients with chronic diseases who are at the highest risk for death and poor outcomes are those with the least access to technology. Are we just deepening the divide?

8

THE DEEPENING DIVIDE

In a digital society, digital rights are civil rights.
FRANCELLA OCHILLO

There are some things in life that you can never let go. You persevere and always question yourself about whether we could have done better. Could *I* have done better? One of these things is the death of my grandmother while in a nursing home. Approximately eighteen years ago, at around 3:00 a.m., I received a call from the skilled nursing facility saying that my grandmother had fallen out of bed and was being rushed to the local community hospital. My grandma, who I fondly called "Biji," was probably one of the strongest women I have ever known. She was the matriarch and the backbone of the family and lived the last several years of her life with me.

Biji had long-standing chronic obstructive lung disease and mild diabetes, beyond which she was doing pretty well. She was a resoundingly healthy eighty-five-year-old who managed all her activities of daily living quite well, with little to no assistance. About a week prior, she had experienced a seemingly concerning flare-up of her underlying respiratory condition, and her primary care physician had admitted her to the neighboring community hospital in suburban Boston for a quick course of antibiotics and steroids. She recovered in four days and was redirected to the nursing home for a few more days of antibiotics and physical therapy. It was her first day at the facility, and I had visited her earlier that evening. She was in a semiprivate room, and her neighbor across the curtain had been there for more than two months and was bedridden. In comparison, Biji was the pinnacle of good health. The intent was for her to stay a couple of days, gain some strength, and come back home. That night, at around 2:15 a.m., the nursing staff heard a loud thud from her room.

Per their report, Biji had climbed out of bed and was making her way to the bathroom, where she slipped and hit her head on the concrete floor. She died instantly.

Within fifteen minutes of the call I reached the hospital, where she had already been pronounced dead. A life prematurely ended. There are many things that went wrong here: the absence of remote video monitoring, the undetected stepping out of bed, the fall, the lack of an elder-friendly environment coupled with suboptimal monitoring, staffing, and care. What happened to Biji, though, is not uncommon. It was not the first time this had happened and certainly was not limited to this facility. I believe this is still a daily occurrence across the country. It was not okay eighteen years ago and is certainly not acceptable today. The presence of video-assisted monitoring with the aid of wearables and passive sensors integrated in the bed, surrounding walls, and furniture can preclude and mitigate any similar unfortunate circumstances. Staffing and skilled nursing are still in short supply, and this is where technology can help anticipate, avert, and potentially avoid similar incidents.

AGING IS A DISEASE

The nation's changing demographics and increasing proportion of elderly patients continues to weigh on the health care system. It is terrible that in the penultimate years of our lives, care delivery does not remain equitable. The have-nots and the disenfranchised become the have-nothings. As we get older, we carry a higher burden of chronic diseases. This is further compounded by infirmities, cognitive issues, and frailties. Many of these get labeled as social issues and are left untended. Getting old is really tough. I sometimes feel that aging is not as physiological as we claim it is, but more of a disease. What makes it even more challenging is that even though the need for access increases with age, it's not always easily available.

Enter telemedicine. Telehealth technologies give us the opportunity to level the playing field and allow us to provide timely interventions that can mitigate emergencies and avert hospitalizations. These may enable the elderly to stay in their own homes, remain independent longer, and avoid care facilities. Telemonitoring platforms are being developed that can monitor the vital signs and physical activity of the elderly living alone. These platforms include a variety of sensors that are user-friendly and automated—to measure weight, heart rate, blood pressure, oxygen saturations, gait stability, fall risk, and activity. This can include a combination of sensors embedded in chairs, beds, and phones, or motion sensors within the corridors of the house. These send automatic periodic or triggered transmissions to the remote server, where the data is displayed on a clinical portal for clinicians to monitor. Any change in habits, instability, or susceptibility to falls and injury can be dealt with quickly.

Such strategies are scalable but, unless automated, may remain impractical. The elderly population comes with many forms of disabilities and levels of frailty. The need for reliable alerts and limiting false alarms will be crucial. The constant data feed allows for machine learning and developing algorithms that can be reliable across different settings, homes, and clinical conditions. Unfortunately, this technology currently is for only the privileged. It is for us to create the infrastructure toward enhancing health equity for the elderly and other vulnerable populations. The technology is here. Now we need to make it accessible and simple.

The bottom line here is simplicity: a telemonitoring system that is simple to use, not clunky, with plug-and-play installation and an integrated platform allowing for an expanded use of sensors for a variety of chronic diseases. The key features involve telehealth-supported continuous wireless transmission of activity and physiological data that is amenable to analysis and alerts. Such systems enable the integration of health and social care on a single platform. The movement and activity data can indicate that a patient has fallen, capture exaggerated nighttime activity suggestive of a disease flare-up, or identify frequent visits to the bathroom due to a urinary tract infection. I cannot overemphasize the importance of habit data here. Often a simple change in habits may be a harbinger of worse things to come. Some of this is still difficult to quantify and develop algorithms around. But the greater deployment of passive sensors will enable this to become a routine form of remote monitoring in the future. The telemonitoring service allows for the fusion of data from multiple sources and sensors, prioritizing them by an algorithm-derived categorization into levels of urgency or emergency.

The need for reliable alerts and limiting false alarms is key. As stated in the section on sensors, multiple sensors with either an integrated index or with well-characterized algorithms with combined decision rules across multiple parameters have been key to these platforms working well in select populations. Developing robust algorithms that are reliable across different settings, homes, and clinical conditions is key to the success of such an integrated platform. These services seem optimal for the elderly with the most advanced diseases, with a high likelihood of having serious adverse events that could be intervened upon proactively. But as we get better at collecting and analyzing this data and the sensor sophistication is further augmented, this may become common practice across all senior-housing facilities. Getting old may not be as physiological as it is claimed to be, but telehealth and remote monitoring can take away the anxiety of being alone and vulnerable.

A DIVIDE BEYOND AGE

Ashley is a forty-three-year-old woman with heart disease living in Brookline, an upscale suburban neighborhood of Boston. Over the last six months, Ashley has been able to see all her doctors (including me) through virtual video visits. Throughout the pandemic, she has not had to step foot into the hospital environment yet was still provided with all the necessary resources to manage her condition.

Now I'd like to introduce you to Silvia, a thirty-seven-year-old mother of two suffering from the same heart disease as Ashley. Silvia lives with her family in Chelsea, a town just as far away from our hospital as Brookline is, but with markedly different demographics. Unlike Ashley, Silvia has not had the comfort and assurance of virtual visits. Because of her unreliable internet connectivity, Silvia has had to resort to telephone conversations (which are often insufficient) and sometimes even show up in person, despite her concerns about the pandemic.

By way of this pandemic, we have more willingly accepted and implemented the world of virtual health care. Amid the contagion, patients had the opportunity to maintain their necessary care while still limiting their risk of exposure. But not all patients have that privilege. Patients such as Silvia had to keep making trade-offs: Does she take care of her chronic condition, or does she avoid the risk of infecting herself and her family with COVID?

The reality is that much of our population faces the same dilemma as Silvia; in fact, approximately half the US population has a slow or unreliable internet connection. This is much worse in states with many rural residents, such as Montana, where more than a quarter of residents don't have internet access at all, and those who do have the worst internet speed in the nation. In the cardiology practice where I work, more than half the patients were unable to have video visits and had to resort to either telephone calls or in-person visits. Our research work, supported by that of others, has shown that these patients are predominantly from minority groups and have an increased likelihood to be either uninsured or covered by public insurance options such as Medicaid. This contributes to threefold less likelihood of being able to connect with their doctor via virtual video visits. Moreover, if patients do not speak English, there is a fivefold increase in not getting to see their doctor virtually. This reality of inequity constitutes what is known as the digital divide.

DIGITAL INEQUITY = HEALTH INEQUITY

The lopsided damage of this pandemic to the African American, Latinx American, and Native American communities has exposed the long-standing structural racism that exists within the US health care system. Our society and government were built on laws, policies, and practices that have disadvantaged the lives of minorities. The structural discrepancies—across living standards, education, social inclusion, and much more—have resulted in lingering inequities in health care that have left our already disenfranchised patients even more vulnerable.

Hospitalization and death rates in these communities have shocked the world and shown us that the system has done little to improve health care access and the quality of care for the disenfranchised. Delayed diagnosis, suboptimal treatment, and lack of preventative care measures have existed for too long. Coupled with this insufficient access to care, Black and brown Americans with low median household incomes living in high-density neighborhoods have become the perfect hosts for the COVID-19 virus. Moreover, many individuals from these marginalized groups have comorbid conditions such as high blood pressure, diabetes, and heart disease that make them all the more vulnerable. Moreover, Black and brown communities fill most of the essential and frontline jobs that cannot be done remotely. This includes health care, transportation, food supplies, waste management, and so on. With continuous environmental exposure, lack of sufficient care, and the multitude of other social inequities that affect them, minority communities are consistently more vulnerable in the wake of the ongoing pandemic.

The worst part of it is that the system has always tried to explain it away, never tried to fix it. Time and again, behavioral, psychological, and cultural issues have been inappropriately propped up as the key reasons for poor health conditions of minorities. And regrettably, there remains an overwhelming ignorance of the everyday actualities that shape the lives of these underserved communities. And now, the digital divide only amplifies these deeply rooted inequities. What we need is digital inclusion. This requires active commitment. This goes beyond internet access and the availability of an appropriate internet-connecting device and refers to promoting digital literacy to enhance the engagement with technology. All clinicians must recognize that a patient's digital literacy is a learned skill, and that the hospital systems they work in must have the ability to promote the acquisition of this skill set among its patient communities.

BRIDGING THE DIVIDE

It's not going to be easy, as there is so much to set right. But we do have to start somewhere, and ensuring universal internet access seems like a good place to begin. We know that unreliable internet access is an important contributor to digital and social isolation, which limits educational opportunities and impedes self-development and wealth generation. All this contributes to the vicious downward spiral etched into the lives of the disenfranchised. This exists in not only rural communities but also inner-city and urban areas with limited resources. Importantly, of the many social determinants (e.g., food, housing, and transportation) contributing to poor health and worse outcomes in minority communities, the digital divide has gained notoriety as a prominent contributor. It is well known that upstream and early interventions in these vulnerable populations can reduce hospitalizations, readmissions, and costs. The journey to ensuring health and digital equity cannot be done with just good intentions and without partners in the community.

Measuring the extent of the crisis and then using data to drive behavior change is always the first step. I think we are already in the drive-change mode. Efforts need to be multipronged, at the federal, state, municipal, community, hospital, clinician, and individual levels. A formidable problem is the lack of broadband connections with high-speed internet access. This is a big challenge to deliver, especially since the internet pipelines are controlled by corporate goliaths such as Comcast, Verizon, and AT&T. They have a for-profit agenda and a corporate culture with a different set of priorities. This is where federal and state regulation with or without incentives is needed to solve the problem. We need a national intervention to standardize the delivery of technology. Like food, water, and electricity, internet access should be a human right.

Just having internet access is not good enough; it must also be fast enough. Connectivity cannot continue to be a barrier. Recently, the Federal Communications Commission has initiated two programs to support telehealth. The Healthcare Connect Fund Program aims to expand telehealth and high-quality internet services to health care facilities beyond just rural areas. The Connected Care pilot program is another program aiming to expand telehealth and mobile-health strategies to underserved, low-income, disenfranchised patients. The intent is to cover 85 percent of costs for broadband connections, related paraphernalia, and information provision. Additionally, statewide initiatives to increase community access to technologies, so that every individual has access to a computer a reasonable distance from their home, will be a step closer to bridging this divide.

Local hospitals and tertiary centers need to show leadership. Their efforts at prioritizing and correcting the inequity need to become more than lip service or photo ops. Incentivizing culture change needs to be a part of the mission—one that is fully resourced and accompanied by structured payment models to ensure the durability of the culture change. There can be no ambivalence here, and there needs to be support and a mandate from the highest rung of leadership within hospitals. Rather than setting up expensive ambulatory-care centers in areas with high-end commercial insurance, putting up health care kiosks with digital access in the community centers, schools, and libraries of disenfranchised communities needs to become a priority, as does setting up hot spots for free Wi-Fi access in multiple locations within rural or inner-city regions to facilitate access to health care, education, and opportunities for upward social mobility. At the individual clinician level, a steady feed of metrics to maintain heightened sensitivity to existing inequities and personal accountability toward individualizing care to mitigate them are equally important as national policy changes.

There is no better handheld computing system than the ever-progressive smartphone. In a recent survey, almost half of Americans stated their preference for using cell phones when communicating with their doctors. Makes sense, as it is a user-friendly tool that is always at hand. More than 85 percent of Americans already have a phone, and notably, Black and Hispanic Americans own smartphones at identical rates to white Americans. It is through this device that we may be able to build bridges across the divide.

We are all connected with one another. COVID-19 has shown us that we cannot separate our health from those around us. If we want to stay healthy, we need to improve the overall health of our society. We need upstream interventions, ones that will help address many of the social determinants of health and systemic inequities. Without digital equity, we cannot achieve health equity. The momentum from the pandemic can help us reinvent health care at the population level and bridge this divide with the disenfranchised. We need to pause and take a step back to see how telemedicine and digital advances can be applied across all communities and all types of homes. One early intervention being put into place is the distribution of free (returnable) iPads coupled with a digital access coordinator program serving to address the gaps in digital literacy. Looking ahead, we should not proceed with the intent of backfilling the gaps later but make fixing this inequity a proactive forward journey. This way we won't have to spend the next several decades righting the wrongs of the present one.

VIRTUAL GLOBAL HEALTH EQUITY

Having spent the first thirty years of my life in India and also working in rural hospitals, I can state with certainty that "under-resourced regions of the world" will need something completely disruptive to ensure and enhance health equity. Improving care delivery in the low- and middle-income countries facing issues with short staffing, limited resources, variable quality, and inadequate access to care is a worthy challenge to take on. Clinical medicine in many less-developed parts of the world remains just a diagnostic science, with no therapeutic options available. During my early years of training at David Sassoon General Hospital in Pune, India, one's proficiency in medicine was determined by ascertaining the right diagnosis; when it came to treatment options, the discussion was speculative and theoretical at best. Things have gotten better now, but not so everywhere. It is here that the smartphone and telemedicine offer a unique opportunity for change. Connectivity and the increase in computing power create an opportunity to enhance this global health initiative.

First, any new technology uptake is determined by the demographics, cultural underpinnings, lifestyles, and disease or biological susceptibilities within a population. Telehealth is the first step and sensor strategies the next, but the rapid evolution of the technology, accompanied by an evolving, chaotic world of predictive analytics fueled by AI, can add another layer of complexity. Providing the right set of incentives, with the goal of global health equity, while proactively predicting and mitigating any negative downstream impact on stakeholders will be essential to getting these noble efforts off the ground.

This becomes even more imperative when we begin to examine the prospect of transforming global health. If there is a time and a willingness to do this, it is now. A pandemic has not only exposed local and regional inequities, but it has also brought forth the raging differences between the privileged and less-developed countries.

This will not be easy, but that makes it even more worthwhile. Many, if not most, of the health systems in low- and middle-income countries lack the appropriate infrastructure to regulate, monitor, and ensure high-quality clinical care. Add to this the lack of technology, and this may make implementation and regulation even more challenging. But if technology is integrated within the lifestyle and daily use (like the smartphone), then we have a winner. The issues of patient privacy, human ethics, literacy, liability, and data security will remain challenges and will be different within each community. Especially as this kind of care crosses national and international borders, having some rules around the provision of clinical care will be necessary. Using the COVID pandemic and the future risk of recurrent virus-related surges as leverage help make the case for making health care equitable.

Why the inertia, and what will it take to edge this forward? Leadership, political will, and a sense of urgency coupled with prioritization of such global strategies are central to making this successful. I think we have all begun to realize how interconnected we are, and a new "bug" in a low- or middle-income country can easily find its way across the rest of the globe and vice versa. Lifestyle practices and high incidence of heart disease have become a return gift from the high-income countries to the rest of the world. We are all one. There is give-and-take commercially, intellectually, and in disease. Sensor-backed AI-based solutions will enhance that interconnectivity and allow us to look after each other and behave like a larger global community, rather than the silos that exist today. We have already begun to see the dissemination of virtual medical care across the US to communities stricken by calamities, and to other countries enmeshed in war.

Recent reports have suggested that almost 85 percent of the world's population (5.1 billion people) has access to 3G or higher mobile broadband coverage. This extended coverage into low-socioeconomic-status households and rural areas enables telehealth-assisted delivery of health care to regions with limited resources, all via a handheld smartphone. This can take care of access issues and associated health care costs in regions where transport and travel themselves are significant barriers to care. It goes without saying that this will further heighten the relevance of implantable and wearable sensors. Universal health care coverage systems must become a way of life, as more and more people travel and stay for long durations outside their domicile country. And then we have almost everyone striving for low-cost solutions to survive a cost-escalating environment of new drug and device discovery accompanied by spectacularly high prices. Sensors and apps on our phones are low-cost strategies that can capture a spectrum of data, either from the clinical encounter or periods of wellness surveillance in between visits.

There are many stakeholders here: the patient; the provider; the hospital system; and the local, regional, national, and international regulatory bodies. Importantly, the right suite of apps and sensors will need to end up with the right patient and provider. Every practice will be different and will need to adapt to local needs. The connectivity will enable local physicians, as well as those from across the globe, to work together to provide the best service. The contractual requirements of local governments, the medical industry, distant, renowned academic medical centers, and their physicians will evolve. There will be many challenges along the way, but if we are proactive, we can begin to pave the path for global health equity.

9

DIGITAL PRIVACY—AN OXYMORON?

Privacy with medical information is a fallacy. If everyone's information is out there, it's part of the collective.
CRAIG VENTER

I have known Betsy for the past fifteen years. She is sixty-three years old and was referred to me for a second opinion after experiencing an episode of syncope (loss of consciousness). This was an unheralded episode of fainting with no clear signs or symptoms preceding the event, which occurred while she was stepping off the curb to board a bus. It was unclear whether the fall was mechanical—she could have just slipped and fallen—or whether was there an underlying medical condition contributing to this event. I put her through a battery of tests to look for heart-rhythm-related issues or any structural problems with her heart, essentially to rule out any possibility of this happening again. Everything turned out to be negative. A Holter, echocardiogram, MRI, stress test, tilt table test—all negative. As a form of exaggeration, it is something we call a million-dollar workup. Despite not having any major cardiac issues and never having had a recurrence of her loss-of-consciousness episode, she continues to follow up with me on an annual basis. It is usually a "Hi, hello, how're you doing?" kind of a conversation, but we hit it off well, and to this day she continues to stay my patient.

Betsy struggled with her weight for many years until she started developing knee issues along with a recent diagnosis of type 2 diabetes. She was motivated to lose weight and began looking for apps to help her to do so, and she fell in love with the MyFitnessPal app. She became profoundly diet and exercise conscious and began losing weight. It was her "endorphin release," and every time she came into the clinic, she would pull out her phone and begin scrolling through screens to show me how cool the app was. She would reiterate that it had changed her life. She had lost weight and managed to keep it off. Every time she ate something she should not have, she was quick to do a calorie count and assess her need for exercise to combat the extra calories, and she would get to work. She had a regimen, and she was doing well. She had lost thirty-two pounds and felt the best she ever had in her life.

And then the breach happened. One hundred fifty million accounts (including hers) were hacked. Betsy was livid; her privacy had been invaded, her trust eroded, and she had lost confidence in reengaging with the world of mobile health. The hackers had their usernames, passwords, and email addresses. This remains the biggest issue with apps and digital devices: securing health technology is challenging, and the threat from malware and hackers remains a real and present danger. If it is fitness data, one may not be that worried, but the moment we begin talking about more sensitive genetic information, then that is a problem. The data being generated with digital wrist devices are usually aggregated across the population for research purposes, and hence the extent of harm at the individual level is limited. Again, if there is personal and genomic information, then the whole equation of risk and liability changes. And then there is a library of mHealth apps collated by the National Health Service in the UK in an attempt to ensure that all these meet the highest standards of privacy and safeguard sensitive, health-related information. A review of these apps from the Imperial College revealed some disturbing findings: approximately 20 percent of them lacked privacy standards, and two-thirds did not use encryption when sending personal identifying information over the internet. It may not surprise anyone that these apps are free or minimal cost and that they use any tactic they can to make themselves sticky and difficult to renounce. The currency here is personal health data. It's not yours anymore. That is the exchange. And that needs to be fixed.

Also, in the United States, these digital devices are not regulated under the Health Insurance Portability and Accountability Act (HIPAA), which governs patient privacy. This allows these companies to gather and sell users' electronic data indiscriminately. There are already health insurance and life insurance companies using digital health solutions to motivate patients to live healthy lifestyles with add-on incentives such as reduced premiums, gift cards for apps, and appliances such as a smartwatch and digital-monitoring tools. There is a fear that, in the future, health insurance companies will deny coverage for individuals who practice unhealthy habits and who may have underlying conditions that are unmasked through these digital devices. This could begin to infringe on personal rights. It also may not be long before there is reverse discrimination, where the insurance companies penalize the patient for not reaching specific goals set for them on their lifestyle-management dashboard.

DIGITAL SPEAK AND TEXTING

Virtual care without an objective clinical assessment strategy is akin to practicing half-baked clinical medicine. You may practice it, but you can never be sure that your clinical judgment is spot on. In the era of telehealth, the physical exam is nearly defunct. To overcome some of this, we now have an array of doctor-assistance apps, which assimilate data from sensors and provide a display of multiple graphs to the doctor to help objectify a virtual visit. It is still unclear what data will be compiled and how much. This can be different for different doctors and subspecialties. As discussed earlier, the digital stethoscope (Eko) can record and transmit lung and heart sounds to the clinician. There are already AI-assisted strategies working on analyzing these to help make a clinical diagnosis. One can keep the transmittal of this digital data simple or add to it a sensor output from a multitude of other sensors embedded within home appliances, security systems, or hospital equipment, all of which provide more granular information about the patient's clinical condition, ambulatory state, ability to perform activities of daily living, and vulnerability to fall or injure themselves. This is considerably more evolved than texting and serves to help the clinician provide patient-centric care in real time.

On the other hand, texting is ubiquitous. It is user-friendly. My eighty-three-year-old mother and many of my octogenarian patients are adept at texting. The Pew Research Center has suggested that greater than 80 percent of adults text regularly and 90 percent of those texts are opened within five minutes on a smartphone. The best thing about texting is that it still seems nonintrusive. You can choose to ignore it. Texting offers access and scalability across space and different time zones. Like many of my colleagues, I don't use voice mail anymore. As an interventional electrophysiologist, I can be tied up in procedures or surgeries for six hours at a time, so I ask my patients to text me and tell them not to expect an answer back in a hurry, but surely by the end of the day. Obviously if there is an emergency, they know not to text but to page the emergency line instead. There is data to confirm that clinician access has been shown to enhance sustained engagement and is associated with improved satisfaction and outcomes. Just the notion of having access to the doctor provides solace to patients and has on many occasions averted the angst of an unnecessary visit to the ER. Texting is particularly helpful in the post-discharge period to keep the connectivity via a digital dialogue. This helps keep patients educated, reminded, and engaged. It helps reduce readmissions and disease flare-ups.

Notably, texting and other forms of digital communication are useful across a spectrum of clinical situations. Kick Butts is a text-based tobacco-cessation program used to change lifestyle in Walmart employees. Similarly, texting-aided diabetes management programs exist to improve medication adherence, self-care tasks, better ER utilization, and patient satisfaction. These have been shown to reduce HbA1c by 1.05 at six months and ER visits by 20 percent. There is a science to this. Many of these platforms, be they for patient engagement, medication adherence, or physiotherapy, are individualized, with some common frameworks and principles to guide them. This is backed by behavioral science using the IMB (information, motivation, and behavioral) model. For texting to work, the technology needs to click back to the care team and integrate across different care settings. The digital dialogue strategy needs to effortlessly align with existing workflows and care pathways. There are many ways to make this work without overburdening the physician. These texts may be filtered and triaged by an unlicensed specialist to the appropriate clinician. This could well be a registered nurse, the nurse practitioner, or a physician's assistant. Some of this is already finding its way into the care pathway using health care navigators, a new job description gaining traction in the construct of these newfangled disease management platforms. The problem, however, remains one of privacy. It is worth reminding ourselves that texting is still not a HIPAA-compliant way of sharing any sensitive clinical information.

APPS

Currently there are several hundred thousand mobile health apps, and their number continues to exponentially increase. These are commercially driven, with limited oversight from any health care regulatory organization. Data privacy and efficacy are in the back seat, and the forward momentum is about getting users and generating revenue. There are also issues with accuracy and reproducibility of many of the measures. Even though these make it to the market under the guise of wellness tools and avoid the rigor of medical grade approval, we know that many patients are using these wearables to guide their activities. This can be harmful and, in some cases, lead to death.

This is exemplified by the class-action lawsuit filed by the State of California against Fitbit in 2016. Researchers from California State Polytechnic University highlighted that the Fitbit was underestimating the heart rate by approximately twenty beats per minute during moderate levels of exercise when compared to a streaming ECG recording. And if a heart rate monitor is underreporting a heart rate to a cardiac patient using it to gauge their level of exercise, then we have a problem. Patients can overstep and push themselves further, to the extent that it could lead to harm. I always tell my patients, "It is those that exercise too little or too much that keel over." This would be a risk for the latter group. The same is applicable to apps that monitor blood pressure, temperature, oxygen saturations, and so on. If these measures are erroneous, they can lead to significant harm.

The FDA is trying to find a way to keep up with this explosive increase in software development. It launched a software precertification pilot program in 2017 to keep tabs on the safety and effectiveness of software technologies, which will attempt to ensure some regulatory underpinnings while allowing patients to access these innovations. There is no going back, as these apps will transcend from the world of wellness to that of disease. They have the potential to offer patients and researchers large amounts of continuous data with a high level of granularity. It is still unclear how these will integrate into the workflow of clinical practice and into large databases that can be mined to enhance the delivery of precision medicine.

Many apps have been shown to be vulnerable to application programming interface (API) cyberattacks that could allow unauthorized access to patient records, lab results, images, blood work, medications, social security numbers, family details, and other personal information. HealthITSecurity has pointed out that with the increase in mobile health apps during the pandemic, there has been a greater than 50 percent increase in cyberattacks. As much as we value privacy, a counterargument is that sharing information without filters can speed up research. The truth of this has certainly become very clear during the COVID pandemic, where time has been of the essence. There is no time to invest in bureaucracy or try to levy clunky and cumbersome privacy policies. There is a plethora of information about the disease state, clinical and laboratory profiles that we need to share quickly while ensuring the personal and sensitive information is protected. Some of this may apply to the world of apps as we get used to using them, and then maybe backend the regulations. Some of that for sure will happen with virtual care and telehealth. Regulatory bindings on the privacy end of things will initially slow down the pace of adoption and integration with conventional workflow. But once we figure out the right formula and put into place the right template to address the multiple issues, we will be on our way.

PART III

ARTIFICIAL INTELLIGENCE

10

DEMYSTIFYING AI

Is artificial intelligence less than our intelligence?
SPIKE JONZE

Hector's device shocked him at 9:43 p.m. precisely, when he was watching the baseball playoffs. It was a home game, bottom of the eighth inning, and the Red Sox were not doing too well. He had gotten quite used to the unpredictable nature of the game and the lack of consistency of his favorite team over the years. Nevertheless, he could not prevent himself from getting worked up. It was during a swing and a miss that he noticed his heart racing and some light-headedness. He could feel the beginnings of losing consciousness before he received the sudden jolt in his chest. It saved his life.

Hector, a forty-two-year-old retired firefighter, suffered a massive heart attack three years ago. I first met him after the heart attack, when his heart function had taken a big hit and was half of what it should be. Despite medications to strengthen his heart, it had not recovered, and his left ventricular ejection fraction was at 25 percent (normal being greater than 50 percent). Hector's heart muscle was significantly scarred from the heart attack, and it was highly unlikely that it would improve. In fact, the natural history of similar disease states suggested the possibility of a gradual decline over the coming years. I was seeing Hector for his risk of sudden death.

When the heart is scarred, it makes the individual susceptible to developing life-threatening arrhythmias originating from the ventricles of the heart. These malignant heart rhythms, known as ventricular tachycardia or fibrillation, can lead to cardiac arrests, oftentimes with no clear triggers. It is patients with similar kinds of scarred and damaged hearts who are served well by an implantable defibrillator. This is the device Hector had. It typically is implanted in the left upper side of the chest just below the clavicle and under the skin and adjoining subcutaneous tissue. The electronic device is connected with a wire that is snaked into the heart from a venous channel in the shoulder. This lead system picks up electrical signals on a beat-to-beat basis from within the heart, and depending on what the device "sees," it either electrically paces the heart when it goes too slow or shocks the heart if it detects a fast, life-threatening arrhythmia. This is what happened to Hector. He got shocked. When he reached the ER, I was able to place an electronic wand over his device in the left shoulder region and extract data noninvasively. The information showed that Hector had developed spontaneous ventricular fibrillation. The device was able to pick up the electrical signals from his heart, analyze the signals, determine that this was real and life-threatening, then shock his heart back into rhythm all within nine seconds, saving his life. The implanted device was programmed with a form of limited artificial intelligence to pick up and interpret electrical signals and deliver a treatment strategy. This is what we call a narrow form of AI. This already exists and works really well in saving lives.

Narrow forms of AI, defined by the ability to perform a single intelligent task that is confined to a code, have been in our lives for several years. It is general AI (a broader form of AI)—reflective of adaptive intelligence exhibited by humans, where machines can sense, reason, and think like people—that remains elusive. For instance, this could involve conducting tasks as complex as cutting hair, cooking, crossing an overcrowded road, performing surgery, or making a clinical diagnosis. General AI is inherently more sophisticated and can be defined in many ways.

DEFINING AI

For the last fifty years, we have heard that AI will take over our lives in the next ten years. We finally seem to be inching closer to when that prediction time frame may begin to ring true. But let's start by going back in time. Back in the 1950s, Alan Turing first brought up the question "Can machines think?" He went on to conceive and model the development of the artificial neural network of algorithms after the human brain. Within this modeling, the processing and reprocessing of information closely mimicked the flow of information within the layers of neurons and their interconnecting synapses in the human brain.

The father of AI, Marvin Minsky, described AI several decades ago as "the science of making machines do things that would require intelligence if done by men." Simplistically, it is when a computer is able to perform functions that were previously thought able to be performed only by humans. More recently, Amazon Web Services described AI as a field of computer science dedicated to deciphering cognitive problems commonly associated with human intelligence such as learning, problem-solving, and pattern recognition, the intent being not to replace the human decision-making process but instead to complement it. Even though the term *AI* was coined over half a century ago, it took several decades for it to get traction, because of limited computing power. The Electronic Numerical Integrator and Computer (ENIAC), which was the first programmable computer, made in 1945, was a room-size machine with the ability to solve simple numerical problems. Now we have the iPhone 13, which has within it fifteen billion transistors and a processing speed several thousand times faster, and all in your hand.

We see many forms of AI in our everyday life. This could be the ubiquitous virtual assistants (i.e., Alexa or Siri), online and computer algorithms to recognize photos and detect spam, or the refinement of self-driving cars, autopilots, air traffic scheduling, auto trading, and fraud detection. When it comes to repetitive tasks that involve processing large amounts of data and need high speed complemented by consistency, it seems like the perfect setup where AI can help.

What about in clinical medicine? The current demand for "value" in a world of progressive digitization with relentless reams of free-flowing data has created an expectation for immediate personalized care. It is a scenario where only a machine can digest all that data speedily and spit out recommendations that the clinician can quickly put to use. Patient data now goes way beyond what is located within the EMR. In fact, the EMR is only a small component of the big story of a patient's life that can affect the occurrence of disease. There is now an ever-intensifying geyser of information from a multiplicity of sources, inclusive of mobile devices, implanted or wearable sensors, environment, social media, imaging, and genomic and other biomedical data that extend beyond the realm of conventional practice. Data continues to increase, without a parallel increase in the human cognitive capacity. The human brain is unable to handle this data deluge and can be overwhelmed enough to cripple any decision-making. AI serves as a powerful software-engineering fix for large amounts of unstructured data that would make clinical practice resourceful, expedient, and more tailored to the specific patient.

DEMYSTIFYING AI

Even though the boundaries of AI may seem vague and limitless, it is important for us to first demystify this entity and then customize it to our needs. Many AI opponents continue to present AI through the lens of science fiction, promoting a far-fetched dystopian ideology. Some appropriately call it augmented or assistive intelligence, while others recognize it as artificial intelligence. A part of this variance in branding comes from its evolving role in daily life, where it either serves to complement a human role or may entirely replace it. Over the years, AI has acquired many definitions and serves as an umbrella term that includes under it a variety of tools such as machine learning, deep learning, natural language processing, and robotics.

Machine learning (a term thrown around quite frivolously) involves engaging a machine (computer) to learn to perform a task without a preexisting code. In the field of medicine, this is possible through a compilation of a large number of clinical case profiles with a known specific outcome. The machine algorithm works its way through this multitude of case scenarios while continuing to learn and adapt to achieve the goal—that is, to predict the proposed clinical outcome. A well-known example of this is "image recognition," where algorithms, after analyzing millions of pictures, can recognize forms, shapes, patterns, and more. This automated intelligence in imaging and signal processing has already made inroads into the practice of medicine through adroitly categorizing dermatological, radiological, ophthalmological, cancerous, and cardiovascular disease states. Almost every discipline in medicine has now been touched by the potential of machine learning. The simple splendor of machine learning is that one is examining the data without prejudging it. There are no assumptions. This allows for the algorithm to be more accurate for prediction and classification, and more generalizable. Of course, the generalizability is determined by the sources and veracity of the datasets used to generate the algorithm.

Machine learning (ML) can be supervised or unsupervised. The principal difference lies in that supervised learning requires a dataset with predictor variables and labeled outcomes. The outcomes are often dichotomized into binary variables: yes and no, dead or alive, hospitalized or not, among a host of other endpoints for assessing the efficacy of a treatment strategy. The issue with dichotomizing endpoints is that we lose a lot of important information along the way, as nothing in medicine is clearly split down the middle.

Supervised ML is the process of modeling the relationship between independent and dependent variables. It involves teaching the algorithm what it needs to learn to accomplish. It is a form of AI used where the algorithm-specific task can be precisely defined by the data at hand. This could include the use of regression, off-the-shelf machine-learning algorithms such as tree-based methods, or support vector machines. Unsupervised learning is learning without a teacher. Different datasets are provided to the algorithm, which then goes on to find an association of its own. This is the perfect way for finding new drug interactions or clustering patients into groups based on their risk profiles for a prespecified endpoint.

Deep learning is a subfield of machine learning that may include performing more than one specific task. This involves the exploration of data with layers of linear and nonlinear transformation organized in a hierarchical way. The basic building block is an artificial neuron that connects layers upon layers from input features to output targets. Notably, deep learning works from very large datasets of covariates and outcomes; it repeatedly and automatically modifies input data using multiple levels of algorithms, abstraction, and adjustment of weights, until a task is learned. An example of this is the processing of several hundred thousand retinal images to learn about more than just the eye disease. In this case, deep learning shows that a retinal image can be used not only to diagnose diabetic retinopathy but also to identify an individual's gender and age as well as the risk of a heart attack.

Neural networks mimic the human brain. Simply put, the brain is like a general processing unit. Every thought process within the brain generates computer graphics, images of people, animals, and inanimate objects. Neuro-evolution in its highest form is where AI is used to build AI with an evolutionary algorithm. Essentially, this is an algorithm that can continually mutate to solve problems as they manifest. It continues to learn and evolve.

AI can never be humanlike if it cannot understand the language. Natural language processing (NLP) applications (another form of AI) use algorithms to break down the spoken or written word and communicate it back to us. This is something we see and experience on a daily basis through the use of virtual assistants such as Siri or Alexa. NLP's role in health care is most important, especially as we try to navigate away from keyboard and mouse clicks and physician burnout. It can be as simple as an application programming interface (API) of the EMR, where simple voice commands help handle clinic files, audio files, and imaging files and find tests of importance very quickly. The role of NLP in the building of AI-derived solutions is based on the ability to map and configure unstructured text into structured fields within an electronic medical record. This enables the conversion of data from a machine into a communicable spoken language that may help initiate a response. It is a tool that will enhance human decision-making with greater speed at a larger scale while accounting for complex interactions that the human mind may not understand.

Simply put, with the incorporation of AI into everyday medicine, we may be moving away from conventional evidence-based medicine, or medicine as we understood it, and toward algorithm-directed precision-based medicine. This is where the iceberg analogy comes in handy. What is evident above the surface of the sea is the evidence-based component, and everything below and invisible to the eye but unwaveringly contributing to the iceberg body, is true intelligence-based medicine. It's just that we still can't see it or explain it. To be able to make this transition from evidence-based to true intelligence-based medicine, AI must be made explainable. It needs to be demystified.

AI AND MAKING A CLINICAL DIAGNOSIS

Making a clinical diagnosis is a convoluted process that contains many steps. Currently this involves a detailed conversation with the patient to collect facts, performing a comprehensive clinical exam (that is gradually becoming extinct), then coming up with a list of causes for the presenting complaint or illness. Adding imaging and laboratory values can further refine and help establish a diagnosis. This may sound simple enough to break up into binary variables to generate algorithms. But nothing in medicine is clearly binary or simple. It is a continuum, until it is not, which is when we die.

Establishing a diagnosis involves ruling out many closely associated conditions, what collectively comprises the differential diagnosis. Beyond this, clinicians often differ in their final diagnosis for even the same condition. This could be attributed not only to their clinical skill but also to their experience, instinct, and ability to recall knowledge.

The human brain can get overwhelmed by the volume of data and the probable permutations and combinations of the different data points. AI has the power to run infinite simulations and zero in on what is most essential. One such form of AI that is gaining traction is called casual reasoning AI or counterfactual AI. This form of AI works beyond the linear deductions that are baked into associative algorithms used to line up diseases with their symptoms. This tool provides clinicians with a second opinion, opening their mind to another set of possibilities. We know that the mind does not know what it has not seen or is unable to recollect. This form of assistive AI can help clinicians diagnose and treat tough clinical problems that they may not have encountered before. As an example, AI could suggest to the clinician several alternative diagnoses for a simple unrelenting fever. Often, when there is no clear etiology for the fever, we ascribe the cause to influenza or some other form of viral fever. Rare infections like leptospirosis, dengue fever, or Lyme disease (among a host of others) that are not that commonly encountered may be missed. Assistive AI could deliver a list of differential diagnoses in rank order that could ensure we check off all the important boxes and make the right decision, making AI more of a complementary tool. A tool to augment our intelligence, as it is becoming clear that a doctor with an algorithm is much smarter than one without.

Machine learning is about more than just the machine. Intelligent solutions do not just surface within a machine. It requires human intelligence to get it there. Clinical acumen is further heightened through collective intelligence, where humans and machines can work together. Outside of medicine, there are many such examples of collective intelligence that have worked well. Two great examples of this collective intelligence are Wikipedia and Google. Wikipedia is a form of technology-enabled intelligence, where thousands of people all over the planet in incremental ways have contributed to creating a remarkably intelligent product. On the other hand, Google comprises millions of web pages stitched together. Again, a form of collective intelligence, where we type a query into the Google search bar and get an amazingly erudite response. At least most of the time.

TRIP OR TRAP?

Everybody seems to be tripping about AI. It is hyped as this magical entity with infinite promise. However, some think of it as a trap. Erik Brynjolfsson from Stanford University has emphasized that AI and machine learning will become a general-purpose technology akin to electricity or the internal combustion engine. Despite the hype, AI is not ready for daily clinical practice, as many of the use cases have so far been modeled only in a research environment; however, the adoption is growing exponentially, and industry analysis has forecast the AI in health care market to grow from $5.9 billion in 2019 to $31.3 billion in 2025. It is not surprising that seven health care companies making it to the Forbes Top 50 are AI-focused. Interestingly, they have some common themes: drug discovery (Atomwise, Genesis, twoXAR, Recursion), wearable monitoring (Biofourmis), blood pathogen analysis (Karius), and image interpretation (Viz.ai). In the setting of the pandemic, all these are areas of immense topical interest. Some companies are even combining technologies to drive precision medicine. An example of this is Imagia, a Montreal-based company using AI for imaging, banding together with Illumina, using AI for genomics (DNA sequencing and analysis).

So, in medicine, are we tripping or are we trapped in what may turn out to be an unfulfilled promise? It is important to recognize that medicine, like any other industry, faces problems of efficiency, costs, and outcomes, and that AI can play a significant role in addressing these. The health care system is a large, complex environment with multiple levels of interactions. Data constantly comes in from different specialty silos: devices, sensors, laboratory values, blood tests, specimens, imaging, procedural, genetics, social media, and so forth.

For starters, recognizing the heterogeneity and variability of the data and creating the right data architecture will be essential. The more data the better, allowing for enhanced training sets. It is quite clear that there is no AI without machine learning. And no machine learning without data analytics. For the latter, there is a need for the right infrastructure. There is no magic here. Just a good plan, hard work, with well-collected and well-annotated data. The trap here for the health care industry is that it will need to evolve its business model to accommodate the deployment of AI strategies. This will have to come from within and with uniform distribution across different regions, states, and countries. Beyond its impact on the local, regional, or global economy, AI will transform the health care system as it frees up billions of hours of worker productivity, allowing for repurposing and redeploying personnel, while making sure all of them work at the top of their licenses. This will enhance the individual- and collective-value proposition. But how does the culture change start?

11

CREATING THE AI CULTURE

Life is like a landscape. You live in the midst of it but can describe it only from the vantage point of distance.
CHARLES LINDBERGH

I met Victoria for the first (and last) time in the fall of 2019. She was a seventy-three-year-old, strikingly majestic Black woman who had an air of confidence that made it clear to me that she was the matriarch and boss of her family. She was here to see me with her twenty-four-year-old granddaughter Alice, her chaperone for the day. I had been asked by the oncology team to see Victoria for increased shortness of breath and swollen feet, supposedly early manifestations of a weak heart, but she clearly had bigger problems.

That day Victoria was wearing a long-sleeved light-yellow T-shirt imprinted with several smiling faces. Intrigued by her T-shirt and in an attempt to break the ice, I asked her about the faces she was wearing. I was taken aback when she introduced each of the seven faces as her family members (three brothers, two sisters, and two daughters) and began recounting how each of them had died, either of cancer or heart disease. She carried them around with her on this personal journey and said that it gave her faith and strength and continually reminded her to be grateful every day for the time she might still have. She also told me that she was not afraid of going to the other side, as she knew they would be waiting for her. She pointed out that Alice, who was accompanying her today, had herself survived leukemia at the tender age of seven and was studying to be a nurse.

Victoria now had recurrent breast cancer. She'd first been diagnosed twenty-five years ago, received chemotherapy, and since then had had two surgeries with a left breast mastectomy and reconstructive surgery. Her weak heart was most likely a result of the chemotherapy she had received. She was what we call a classic case of the triple whammy: first cancer, now cancer again, then heart failure. She was told that she had a recurrence in her right breast, with evidence of metastases to the lungs and signs of fluid building up around her lungs and heart. She was here on borrowed time. She was very direct in her line of questioning: she wanted to know whether another round of chemotherapy with a weak heart would hasten her death and make her even more uncomfortable. I was not surprised when, at the end of the clinic visit, Victoria made it clear that she was not interested in chemotherapy or in any form of heroics to help her weak heart. She died three months later.

There were so many things here that went beyond my simple understanding of clinical medicine. Why did she have a recurrence after so many years? Could it have been predicted? Could an earlier intervention or detection have saved Victoria from the discovery of metastases all over her body? Was there a way that we could predict which patients would develop heart failure from chemotherapy? Are there simple baseline predictors of chemotherapy-induced side effects? Are there downstream events Victoria's granddaughter might have to face that our current clinical insights cannot see? Why did all her family members have such poor outcomes? Is there an interaction between race, genetics, and cancer that was overlooked, or not detected in a timely fashion?

Can AI help us here? Can AI help us see below the tip of the iceberg to where the vast body of the unknown that constitutes the true body of evidence lies? How does one get one's head around this notion of beginning to use AI? Let's try to break this down.

THE AI CULTURE

Using AI to answer any of these questions that don't involve conventional intellect, and often provide inexplicable conclusions, can create an element of distrust. Medicine is different from the AI used for online banking, customer profiling, or cybersecurity—here, the algorithm can affect life and death. And so, when one doesn't understand the reasoning behind a decision or a diagnosis, it asks for quite a leap of faith. But the time is now, and it behooves us to adopt a flexible and inquisitive mindset. First, some basic questions do need to be answered as one embarks on the AI journey: Is the problem that AI is trying to solve for us appropriate for the data or vice versa? Is the data decent? Is it clean and unbiased? We all know that data collected with inherent biases can lead to a biased outcome, and lack of data, missing data, or corrupt data translates into useless algorithms.

The adoption of AI into daily practice does mandate a huge culture change. Implementing AI means we must rethink the entire business model as well as the culture of the organization. Health care organizations will need to demonstrate regulatory compliance by tracking and explaining AI decisions across workflows while correcting for bias and ensuring positive outcomes. AI-aided care in most chronic diseases will change from the conventional transactional visits every three to six months to one of continuous monitored care. As explained in Part IV, Chapter 17, this could lead to the model of exception-based care, where the patient is called in for an evaluation only by exception, when something amiss is noted via remote monitoring. For this to happen will require a supreme level of confidence in the volume, velocity, and veracity of the data with its integration into the EMR and workflow.

AI can fill many gaps and play many roles, and algorithms already work well for several areas of clinical medicine. This could be in the diagnosis of diabetic retinopathy via evaluation of images of the retina. In this realm, deep learning strategies have evolved to a level that internists don't need the specialists anymore. Aided by AI, they can diagnose and spell out the treatment on their own. It is self-evident that this will help decentralize care and limit the need for care coordination with specialists.

On the other hand, algorithms can risk-categorize patients as they get admitted to the hospital and predict with a high level of accuracy not only the outcome but also the duration of the hospitalization. Beyond this, AI's role in the world of clinical trials, drug development, and basic science is exploding. Computational models are getting to a stage that they help us figure out the more successful drug targets, prioritize interventions, pick better surrogate endpoints, and develop models beyond what the human brain can easily see and imagine. Much of this will no longer be anecdotal.

INTUITION, EMOTION, AND AI

Even though the role of AI in medicine continues to evolve, it cannot compete against human sensibilities. At least not yet. Even though AI may outperform a human mind in generating a comprehensive list of alternative diagnoses, it falls short when it tries to match clinical intuition. Human intuition is based on sensory inputs associated with memories and experiences that are challenging to capture via computing strategies and even more difficult to simulate with an algorithm. The inability to reduce emotion to an algorithm is AI's Achilles' heel when trying to mimic human intelligence. These mathematical algorithms are devoid of feeling and cannot account (at least at this stage) for the emotive end of these decisions or the complexity of the social dynamics around the patient.

AI-aided analytics of verbal and nonverbal cues reflective of a patient's emotional state are being refined. Obtaining this information from active and passive sensors, coupled with analytic tools to deduce emotional or psychological state, will become possible. Tools such as videos and still images to access facial expressions, speech, posture, tics, and so on could help quantify emotion and mood and predict the social interaction. For example, some wearables can track a sudden swing in the heart rate or autonomic function in children with autism, to give a clearer picture of the child's mental state. The latter is possible using a watch that adopts a simpler form of AI, where the watch dial is color coded and quickly changes colors depending on the child's emotional state and the stress they may be experiencing.

An AI vendor, Affectiva, among a host of other, similar start-ups, uses optical sensors and cameras to categorize facial expressions. This, coupled with other objective parameters of autonomic tone and heart rate changes, can help categorize the patient's emotional state. Computer cameras are now able to help diagnose heart-rhythm abnormalities or heart disease changes via algorithms to assess facial flushing and color changes. As one can imagine, the effectiveness of such algorithms will need to be specifically refined across different skin tones, races, and ethnicities. More recently, deep learning software has shown its ability to identify the chronological age of an individual as well as recognize cognitive decline via headshots.

Voice is another human characteristic that reflects the emotional state and can be broken down by natural language processing. AI is useful in voice analyses to measure fear, hesitancy, temper, anger, stress, or pleasure. The focus here is on pace, pitch, and tone, among other subtle assessments. In the near future, AI will help diagnose depression, anxiety, and even manic episodes. This could be done with wearables or the smartphone. These AI analytics using facial expression and speech will become an intrinsic part of telehealth interactions, providing the clinician insights into the emotional state of the patient. As described in an earlier chapter, wearables can give continuous feedback on physiological signals that could also give complementary insight into the patient's clinical or emotional state.

AI AND YOUR DOCTOR

Can AI help choose the doctor best suited for you? Traditional resources used to choose your primary care doctor or even a specialist are hit or miss. Whether these are web-based searches or booklets sent to your front door by your insurance company or randomly scanning the yellow pages, it's almost like a lottery. Web reviews, gradings, and endorsements, alongside online personal recommendations, are mostly biased and often polarized. Commentaries from patients are usually driven by an incredibly positive or negative experience that was compelling enough for them to write. And then there are, of course, the glowing tributes and rosy accolades from friends and relatives. Also, studies suggest that the patient-experience review process is faulty and there is no significant association between a commentary and a doctor's clinical performance. These reviews focus on the niceties of a personal interaction, the front office staff, or telephone responsiveness, but not on clinical outcomes. Moreover, a patient may have a phenomenal experience with their doctor but an abrasive encounter at the checkout counter, and you can rest assured that the entire visit experience will be tainted. That online review for the doctor will not look good.

Pairing of EMRs and AI can help predict which caregiver may best serve a patient phenotype with a particular disease profile. There are analytics data that can provide a better understanding of patient needs, physician attributes, and outcome data. AI can comb longitudinal data and spot patterns of successful relationships and outcomes and make suggestions. AI-driven patient-provider connections may be the way to go for enhancing patient experience, provider satisfaction, and overall clinical outcomes.

AI AND THE TRANSFORMED RADIOLOGIST

Will AI kill the field of radiology? This has been speculated about for a few years and has put a lot of my colleagues in radiology on edge, largely because many of the initial use cases for AI were in imaging. AI-driven image interpretation has been shown repeatedly to be efficient, reproducible, and scalable. Nevertheless, it is still a long way from replacing human expertise. Most AI endeavors are highly focused and specialized. It is mostly a one-trick pony that is very effective in doing what it is trained for but may misdiagnose an outlier condition that the algorithm was not trained to interpret.

Radiologists have begun to lose ground in certain areas. Free online tools such as Chester the AI Radiology Assistant can read and interpret downloaded X-rays. These tools, which enable AI-assisted X-ray reading in seconds while keeping data secure, might erode conventional reporting. They're dedicated to diagnosing congestion, cardiomegaly, nodules, masses, pneumothorax, emphysema, and pleural thickening, and they do so with remarkable efficiency and precision. The impact will be felt soon, as these are scalable across countries with minimal computational costs. The fear that radiology-reading algorithms may not work across heterogeneous populations, however, remains real, as the training dataset may not be entirely generalizable.

But this space continues to explode, and every few weeks, there are algorithms being validated and approved for a variety of tasks. The FDA recently cleared several CT algorithms for pulmonary nodule detection. One of these, for example, is Infervision's deep learning tool for segmenting lung CT scans. Infervision is designed to segment lung CT scans to aid lung cancer programs to uncover small, tough-to-see nodules. This would help to refine and reduce CT reading time, while assuring that a dedicated algorithm will prevent human lapses in recognizing subtle radiological findings of concern. As a result of enhanced AI algorithms, CT and MRI scans may be done in the future without the use of contrast agents, thereby limiting the possibility of kidney injury in some patients. Also, the use of AI has the potential to miniaturize some of the conventional hardware setups for radiology. This would not only mean less space for the MRI scanner (which has a large footprint and needs a dedicated large space), but something that could be compressed and made portable enough to be available at the point of care.

As good as these AI models may be, however, they are unable to participate in a multidisciplinary meeting with patients and other doctors to discuss the nuances of imaging and the implied clinical relevance. Barring that, AI tools will continue to serve as an excellent resource and teaching tool for the inexperienced radiologist and trainee, to help spot subtleties—and it may not be too far from the truth that they could lead to the early demise of a generation of radiologists who are not willing to adapt. The expiration date may truly become a reality for some, especially those who don't learn to use AI.

AI IN DIAGNOSING AND TREATING CANCER

Listening to a friend recount her experience with breast cancer, I considered that AI has made significant strides into the diagnosis and treatment of cancer. Shelley recounted to me how her encounter with breast cancer was one with AI. She said that her mammogram was read using machine-learning approaches, the pathology of her breast lump biopsy was evaluated by an AI algorithm, following which she was started on chemotherapy, and the choice of the medicine was also made with the assistance of an AI algorithm. She is doing well and was grateful that, at every step, she had human interaction in addition to the AI. Although there was a mathematical formula helping make decisions, the final call was the oncologist's and Shelley said she benefited from the best of both worlds. Even though the care may sound transformative, it is important to realize that AI-assisted decision support is purely probabilistic. It calculates the likelihood of the desired outcome depending on the available choices. Many times, there can be several approaches with nearly similar outcomes. And further, AI may not be able to account for the impact of unmeasured sociocultural variables on the desired result. In real life, the decision is usually dichotomous. It is usually a yes or no, a right or wrong. Either you proceed in one direction or another. This is where the oncologist remains indispensable. But will that always be the case?

Treating cancer is exceedingly complex, especially when one begins looking at the different organ systems involved, the severity, and the types of cancer. Add to this the breakneck speed of advancements in genomic information, imaging methods, molecular profiling, and new therapeutics, and one begins to understand why there is so much variance in practice and outcomes across the country. Because of this, the interest in using AI to aid in the day-to-day practice of oncology has become a priority. There are already predictive analytic tools that incorporate the use of genomics risk stratification to support clinical decision-making. These are being used in many ways, including predicting risk for adverse events to select chemotherapeutic agents or in the delivery of value-based care. Although this may seem to work well, it is so important to remember that the generalizability of usage is limited. Much of this still hinges on the sources of data and data integrity.

The American Society of Clinical Oncology (ASCO) is working on this with CancerLinQ, a database of real-world cancer cases from cancer centers and oncology practices across the US. More than one hundred practices have completed the required onboarding to link their EMRs to this common database. CancerLinQ has well over 1.5 million cancer patients in their database. These reflect a fairly diverse cohort: those coming from urban, rural, and suburban settings, as well as those from academic and non-academic, small and large hospital systems. While many programs are adopting the AI trajectory, others have refrained from immersing themselves in the AI Kool-Aid lake.

A quick balcony view of most practices reveals that they use more than a thousand chemotherapeutic regimens and different sequences of drugs, with every physician having stylistic shades and variance in their dosing, sequence, selection, and use of supportive regimens. That's correct—more than a thousand with multiple permutations and combinations of agents. AI in its simplest form as a clinical decision analysis tool can help reduce some of this practice variance while providing individualized care led by evidence. It has the potential to reduce the variability of care and increase compliance with evidence-based decision-making. It always helps to have an objective and quantitative reasoning. The fight to integrate AI-based solutions is on, and within the uncertainty of how this will pan out, there is the promise of better-quality care. This is where IBM stepped in and, in partnership with Memorial Sloan Kettering Cancer Center, launched Watson for Oncology in 2015. The plan was to develop a supercomputer that could become a new diagnostic tool after it processed thousands of medical research papers. The goals were laudable, but it was unclear whether they were realistic.

WHAT HAPPENED TO WATSON?

Medicine is complex, and oncology even more so. For AI to work in oncology requires deep learning from large multispecialty databases, datasets, and guidelines. Computational reasoning is then used to apply this knowledge to a specific and mostly unique case. The intent was for the supercomputer Watson to store and index literature, protocols, and patient data. It was to learn continually from test cases with encouraged supervised learning from experts with the goal of facilitating decision-making and selecting treatment options.

Watson may be great for *Jeopardy!*, but it failed miserably in oncology. There are several reasons for that.

The data in cancer was complex and especially messy and filled with gaps when it came to genetic data. But a bigger concern is that there is more to AI assistance in cancer diagnosis and treatment than just data completeness. Cognitive computing works well for late-stage cancer but fails in its ability to help with early stages, probably because in its early stage, cancer requires more of an uncharted, individualized approach. To highlight this point further, a recent study showed that there was a high level of concordance in treatment recommendations between Watson and physicians for late-stage lung cancer with metastases, but not so in the early stages of the disease, likely because in many situations the patient-doctor relationship and shared decision-making influence the final choice of therapy. Multidisciplinary teams consist of oncologists, surgeons, radiologists, radiation-oncologists, pathologists, palliative care specialists, and social workers. There is a lot of complexity here, and the team-based approach seems indispensable. And again, that is not AI's fault of reasoning; it's just the dearth of clear pathways and the data-free zones for every cancer subtype that is further variegated by demographics, social situations, comorbidities, and personal preferences. Add to this the variance in national medical guidelines, licensing of recommended drugs and treatment, insurance coverage, and compliance with screening protocols.

AI or no AI, I think Shelley—every patient—needs the warmth of a physician interaction when they may be dealing with a life-threatening disease. No computer by itself is going to cut it. The integration of computers to help with efficiency of decision-making and reducing practice variance is not front and center for a patient dealing with cancer. The patient's primary interest is in the care they are receiving. Is it the best possible care, and how well does the doctor truly understand their problem?

AI IN THE PHARMA WORLD

Earlier this year, a patient of my colleague, who was operating in the procedure room next to me, had a catastrophic crash at the end of the procedure. The patient was a seventy-three-year-old male undergoing a catheter ablation for atrial fibrillation. This is an invasive procedure that involves heating tissue within the atrium of the heart, where the circuits that cause atrial fibrillation originate. During this four-hour procedure, the surgeon places several catheters and a camera inside the heart. These are snaked up into the heart via the femoral veins from the groin. The surgeon makes a hole with a needle between the right and left atrium so that he can then thread the ablation and mapping catheter into the left atrium, where much of the procedure is performed. There are many places that things can go wrong, right from the needle access to the femoral veins to the transseptal puncture, which involves puncturing the interatrial septum between the left and right atrium. One danger is accidentally puncturing the aorta or slipping outside the heart, both of which can be clinical disasters. Another is perforating the heart during the burning and freezing, causing a stroke. As proceduralists, we are always working with the fear of making a mistake or having a complication while trying to do our best. One of the primary precautions we undertake to prevent a stroke is to keep the blood thin by administering an anticoagulant so that no inadvertent clots form during the manipulation of the catheters in the heart. Once we are done with the procedure, we have to reverse the blood-thinning effect so that we can pull the catheters out of the heart and femoral veins with no bleeding complications, especially in the groin area. To do this, we administer a chemical agent called protamine, which reverses the anticoagulant effect. It was at this juncture, when my colleague gave the patient protamine, that the patient had a severe anaphylactic reaction to the medication. His blood pressure crashed and was unrecordable, and his heart rate accelerated to the 180s.

Fortunately, the patient was on a ventilator during the procedure, so respiratory status was kept stable. Such a dramatic event can have a significant impact on the overall outcome. The patient can have a stroke, a heart attack, or even multiorgan failure. After you spend hours to keep the procedure safe, you can have a near calamity on hand. This patient was in a monitored setting, so my colleague could quickly administer the appropriate medications to counteract this allergic reaction, and after a few hours of intensive care monitoring, the patient recovered completely. This is what we call a near miss, something completely preventable. If we had known that he was going to have an allergic reaction, then several different mitigation strategies could have been put in place.

This is where AI could have helped in arming us with the information of this danger. It's a rare risk, and no one could have suspected this reaction, as the patient was not on any medications that could potentially cross-react with protamine or increase the possibility of this near-fatal reaction. An AI algorithm that considers clinical covariates, genomic factors, and other black-box interactions that we may not understand at this stage could have helped prevent this near-death event. A nationwide database of protamine reactions would allow machine-learning tools to risk-stratify patients pre-procedurally, so that this 1 in 1,000 gamble is significantly reduced or even eliminated. This is one place where AI will chisel and shape the future of predicting and preventing drug reactions and interactions.

Developing drugs is expensive and unpredictable. Oftentimes scientists spend many years in developing a drug thought to be mechanistically useful, only to determine at the very end of the investigative process that it may have significant side effects. Many of these toxic effects manifest at the end of a long, expensive clinical trial, and the drug development has to be scrapped. Millions, sometimes billions, of dollars are lost as a result of these late-stage clinical trial failures, especially if the drug has already tested well in the phase I and II clinical trials. The hope is that AI might help solve this problem. Recent work from the University of Oxford has shown that a machine-learning algorithm may be useful in providing an expectation of adverse events. For this study, a curated dataset of molecular profiling of more than one thousand drugs and nearly ten thousand samples was used. Beyond such investigational work, there are companies (e.g., AI Therapeutics, Healx Ltd., and Pharnext) leveraging AI to optimize the drug-discovery process through decreasing the time to discovery, predicting toxicity, and improving productivity. Not only that, but AI can also help in drug repurposing, finding new indications for an already approved drug. Examples of this include sildenafil for pulmonary hypertension, which is now also used for erectile dysfunction, and remdesivir, which was originally used for treating the Ebola virus and went on to receive emergent FDA clearance for COVID-19. The concept of digital twins has made significant inroads within the pharmaceutical sector. This virtual replica enables the simulation of potential treatments and assessment of interactions with drugs and disease before administering any chemical to a human. These personalized computational models have already had some success in cardiovascular diagnostics and insulin pump controls. More recently, there are scientists building digital twins of the human immune system, which would be pivotal in the development of new drugs and fighting off autoimmune diseases.

There are several other arenas where AI can influence the pharma world. Machine learning can help assess and forecast the use of medications on a large scale, not just foretell shortages. It may help in understanding the pattern of practice and thereby instruct innovative approaches toward its use. AI has already proven its role in pinpointing defects or contaminations and helping execute the recall of drugs. Two recent recall examples are valsartan for high blood pressure and metformin for diabetes—both were noted to have carcinogenic contaminants (from specific manufacturers) and quickly withdrawn from the market. Beyond this, AI can help provide oversight to prescribing patterns and single out suspicious activity. This has played an important role in the opioid crisis by providing pivotal information regarding local, regional, and national distribution of prescriptions, and helping to home in on practices and physicians abusing their privilege. Similar AI tactics can study and predict the use of other seemingly expensive drugs and thereby play a role in promoting value-based care.

BARRIERS TO AI IN CLINICAL PRACTICE

One of the principal barriers to AI getting a stronger foothold is the lack of data completeness or accuracy. A busy clinician will always cut corners, especially when it comes to data entry. I personally find it extraordinarily challenging to be meticulous with data entry into the electronic medical record. Especially on a busy clinic day, trying to spend time adding every little detail related to my patients' medications, personal habits, or new allergies is tiresome. I do not have the time to ensure that every aspect of the EMR I have interacted with is clean and accounted for and research worthy. Even within my own subspecialty, I often don't have time to pay attention to the subtle nuances of disease classification. I may incorrectly label a patient as paroxysmal atrial fibrillation, when he or she may actually have persistent atrial fibrillation, the difference in categorization driven by the duration of the atrial fibrillation episodes and whether they are self-limiting. In the daily hubbub of a busy outpatient practice, I am not thinking of research or datasets. My focus is on the patient and ensuring I have made the right treatment choices; very often this classification may not affect my immediate decision but could surely affect one coming from an algorithm derived from data in the EMR.

Hiring someone to go in and clean up the data entry after each patient interaction for the multitude of patients seen across the practice may be impractical and prohibitively expensive. We need a seamless, intelligent way of acquiring data, as much as we need one to process it. Missing data in contemporary practice is common. Information related to emergency room visits, admissions to hospitals outside the system, and disease exacerbations (monitored and treated over the phone) rarely find their way into electronic medical records. Besides data acquisition, its validation and veracity are as important. Otherwise, crappy data inputs result in crappy outputs. Further, the impact of bias on the algorithms resulting from the exclusion of socially disenfranchised and underrepresented communities is one worthy of a much longer discussion (see next chapter).

At the same time, institutional data may not be generalizable. It seems obvious that a disease-specific algorithm generated at Tata Memorial Cancer Hospital in Mumbai for a type of oral cancer would not be generalizable to the same disease subset of patients treated at Dana-Farber Cancer Institute in Boston. Principal causes for this could be explained by different data sources, different etiologies, different clinical profiles, different therapeutic approaches, and the less-understood ethnic variance in drug metabolism. Also, risk assessment calculated one time at baseline is not meaningful enough, especially as risk is dynamic and always changing over our lifetime.

Predictive models need large datasets with objective evaluation continually interspersed during the entire clinical course. This should also include information on patient experience, appointment cancellation, nonadherence to medications, and relapses. Unfortunately, EMRs do not have this data embedded within their framework to enable their use in emerging predictive models. To err is human; we all miss appointments, forget to take our medicines, expose ourselves to circumstances that put us at risk for infections, or even run out of supplies. How does one account for this missing data, which could have been instrumental in leading to the endpoint being evaluated by the algorithm? What may be considered a *failure* of therapy may be due to *lack* of therapy. And it is self-evident that if a clinician were to have a single situation of being let down by an algorithm, there would be an instantaneous loss of faith. One incorrect interpretation or suggestion from the algorithm can be the start of disregarding any subsequent AI recommendations. In addition, algorithms deteriorate over time. Especially if they are not continuously updated with new experiences and data, they can go off the rails and deliver faulty advice. Medical providers have already seen some of this algorithm corrosion within sepsis-prediction models in intensive care units.

The biggest problem is that data everywhere remains siloed, hoarded by businesses and academic institutions under the pretext of competition and the desire to stay ahead. The data is locked away in incompatible computer systems that remain barricaded by politics. Even though these barriers are breaking, the process remains slow and filled with distrust. Some of that skepticism originates from the unfulfilled promises of Watson in delivering personalized plans for patients with cancer and other disease states. Or the colossal failure of the Google flu tracker in predicting outbreaks before they occur. The pandemic nevertheless has served to catalyze interest in AI and its role in the practice of medicine. AI-driven predictive analytic tools inclusive of clinical and imaging data have served to provide the diagnosis of COVID-19, even before the results of the conventional nasopharyngeal swabs are back from PCR testing. The barriers are dropping but not fast enough, and that may cost lives. We may not be there yet, but surely we are making strides in the right direction.

12

LAZY, STUPID, BIASED, OR SMARTER?

Data is the new oil.
CLIVE HUMBY

"Are there any more unrecognized confounding factors? Have you made sure you are not missing any clinical variable or data point that could impact the outcome of your analysis?" Thus would Marty Larson, a senior statistician at the Framingham Heart Study, prod me during my two years of research there. While studying association or causation, including relevant covariates in the analysis is important so one can adjust for them. The Framingham Heart Study is the longest ongoing prospective epidemiology study in the world. Started in 1948, it was well ahead of its time, as at that time, besides collecting symptoms, signs, and disease information, researchers also collected lifestyle information. Subsequently, in the mid-1990s, they were able to add genomic data of more than three generations of patients' follow-ups to further enrich the database. The Framingham Heart Study is best known for the discovery of the risk factors for heart disease and has significantly affected the practice of cardiovascular medicine. This was all done when computational power was only a fraction of what it is now. Again, the depth and the breadth of the database, despite being among the best in the world, were just a fraction of the size of the databases we deal with now. As good as the research was then, it was only as good as the data available at that time. The data was rigid rather than free-flowing and certainly nowhere near as voluminous as it is now. But it was an amazing start that has changed the way we live our lives and has certainly had a huge impact on worldwide health policies and reducing the incidence of cardiovascular disease.

I always got it wrong. My hypothesis was good, but my ability to predict the strongest association between the clinical covariates and the outcome was invariably erroneous. Part of it was that I could not anticipate the subtle interactions that the computing program was taking into consideration between these different variables. The algorithm in the statistical package then created a rank order of the different clinical variables that predicted risk and poor outcome. When I began looking at relatively less-understood things such as the autonomic tone, which is a measure of the brain-heart connection, I was surprised by the results. The autonomic tone, which I described in more detail in the previous section on sensors, is quantified by a measure called heart rate variability. The brain-heart interaction is associated with a heart rate that is constantly varying with respiration, emotion, exercise, and so on. This variability can predict death. Previous research had shown a strong association of this measure of autonomic tone with diabetes, age, medications, and other clinical factors.

Interestingly, in 1998 (the year of the Framingham Heart Study's Golden Jubilee), when I got access to the genomic data, it was quite intriguing that a significant part of our heart rate variability was explained by our home environment and genetics, almost comparable to the part explained by disease and other clinical determinants such as age and gender. So what may appear relevant today will become less relevant tomorrow as more data accrues, explaining away previous associations. As modern datasets begin to include environmental factors, social media, phone usage, sleep patterns, emotional state, and other forms of unconventional data, it might explain away some of the associations we thought we understood. Handling all this data and making sense of it is where AI comes into the picture.

DATA AND DISEASE

A large part of medicine remains subjective and qualitative. And despite being driven by science, it remains an art. Making a diagnosis and a decision is never easy. Every single variable or data point that we need to examine and treat must be put into the context of the whole human body, during both wellness and disease. Every decision made is a synthesis of this information, which is further aided (or maybe complicated) by research being added to our list of unread literature. We take in the data. We digest it, then use the laws of probability to help guide us in our choice of diagnosis and therapy. Evident lack of uniformity in this decision-making process and the variability in the final choice of therapy become loosely garbed under "physician discretion." The inconsistency in outcomes within regions and individual physicians within the same practice is striking and reflective of this variance. So how does AI fit into this equation? What are the steps we must take to break down the hurdles of adoption?

IBM has developed an AI ladder that is quite applicable to every subspecialty service under the health care umbrella. The stepladder highlights the different steps to make AI operational. First, make data collection simple and accessible. Second, organize the data so it is prepped and ready for analytics. Third, build and scale AI with trust and transparency, and fourth, operationalize AI throughout the organization. This would involve an interplay of collective intelligence resulting from hundreds of machines and humans working together with speed and scale across the health care system. The ultimate goal is to use data to develop algorithms that may influence care and prevent disease—algorithms that could predict the onset of chronic diseases such as Alzheimer's, diabetes, heart failure, lung cancer, leukemia, and psoriasis, among others, so they could be prevented.

The most influential science exists now at the interface of molecular science, genomics, proteomics, sensors, and social data backed by highly efficient computational approaches. All these sources collectively coin one of the most overused terms these days: Big Data. This is further defined by the three *V*s: Velocity, Volume, and Variety. To this one could add another important *V*, Veracity. Velocity reflects the speed of data acquisition and processing and volume the amount of information; variety refers to the different sources and channels for producing Big Data, and veracity is indicative of the data's accuracy. Accruing this requires a significant measure of collaboration between the computational data scientists, physicians, and researchers bringing together their work as the adhesive between distinctive programs, asking different questions with varying levels of intellectual inquiry. Within the sway of this data lies the power to innovate, discover new therapies, and stomp out disease and disparities across the globe.

When we talk about the source of data overload, it becomes one of perspective. Physicians often feel slighted if they are told by a machine what they should be doing. I know for a fact that many clinicians react adversely and often with expletives unfit to report. Almost every time a clinician is halted during their interaction with the EMR for an additional click to respond to a clinical decision analysis tool recommendation, it is met with an outburst of curses. During an interactive lecture at a recent symposium for cardiologists, I asked a large group of specialists looking after patients with heart failure if they preferred to deal with data overload or volume overload. Volume overload was the unanimous response. To explain this further, heart failure physicians are constantly managing patients with failing hearts that are vulnerable to accumulating fluid when the pumping action of the heart is diminished. There is limited forward flow, reduced perfusion of the kidneys, and consequently retention of fluid, which is typically called volume overload. This volume (fluid) overload then needs to be expertly managed by addressing lifestyle factors such as salt and liquid intake as well as meticulous adjustment of their medical regimen. Each of these patients is usually on at least ten different medications. So not an easy job, but one that cardiologists love doing and are very good at.

I then asked them if they would be able to do this for several hundred of their patients with the same level of individualized attention. The answer was a resounding no, of course—because now the volume overload also becomes a data overload. Tracking hundreds of patients with brittle heart failure that can quickly decompensate and need hospitalization is challenging. If you gave these dedicated cardiologists continuous data to peruse on each of these patients, they would find it useful but overwhelming. But if this data were reviewed, analyzed, then signaled out to the doctor only when it was out of range, it would help prioritize and individualize care. It would, in fact, make their life easier and help provide superior care. More data is better, provided it is backed by intelligence that works. Clearly data is the new oil, but it needs to be clean, relevant, interpretable, and actionable.

DATA, VALUE, AND VARIANCE

You will hear this more than once and may also have experienced it: patient care in the United States is fragmented, complex, and expensive. This is also the case in many other places across the world. The big question we face: Can we make it more uniform and high value?

We know how to cluster patients to find meaningful direction and new therapies, but can we cluster clinical providers to figure out ways of reducing this variance in care? Getting data on providers is easy; one can get this through the analysis of social networks, insurance processing, and Medicare claims data. Machine learning can help extract information on the communities providing care, allowing a peek at cost and quality of care. We can examine and potentially modify patterns of provider behavior. This can also help ferret out low-value services and practice variance, both of which are significant contributors to the unsustainability of modern medical practice.

When we look at the ubiquitous EMR, we recognize that it is a static warehouse updated at a planned or unplanned patient evaluation. Even in the absence of constantly streaming information, the data points from the EMR alone can be staggering. Very superficially, the data collected includes demographics, social habits, family history, physical examination, allergies, diagnoses, procedures, medications, laboratory results, vital signs, symptoms, hospitalizations, tests, outpatient visits, provider notes, and so on. This is without including lifestyle, genomics, social media, and wearables data, which may actually contribute more toward understanding disease prediction and risk-factor mitigation. With changing demographics and patients living longer, there will be more data. As we collect more data, it is important that we consider what computer programmer and science fiction writer Daniel Keys Moran has stated so well: you can have data without information, but you cannot have information without data. We must be able to understand what matters and what doesn't. But we don't know what we don't know, and that is where the hope of AI lies.

Let's use the case of routine surveillance colonoscopies in patients above the age of seventy-five. Hundreds, perhaps thousands, of these are done daily and annually in the US. But does it really make sense to do them? Are they cost effective, and does the risk-benefit ratio make sense? Simply put, the risk-benefit ratio here is inverted: patients in this subgroup are at a higher risk of intestinal injury, dehydration, low blood pressure, and fainting. These risks need to be juxtaposed with the risk for colon cancer. It makes more sense to individualize this decision rather than have a rigid population-based approach. There are many other examples of waste from similar redundant practices.

OptumLabs—an open collaborative center for research and innovation—and its data warehouse have already been using algorithms to process claims data to help identify these low-value services, some of which may range from chest X-rays prior to surgery and MRIs for back pain. Every patient in the most stable clinical condition with no cardiac or respiratory disease gets a routine chest X-ray prior to a surgical or interventional procedure. This habitual reflex occurs every day. I order them myself. There is no particular scientific basis for this; it's more of a habit. Or something we might call practicing defensive medicine—just in case we might miss some lurking pulmonary condition that may contribute to a bad outcome of the procedure. It is unclear whether this translates into any form of clinical benefit. The additive cost is humongous, and it is here that AI might help us parse value and facilitate more directed and individualized recommendations for investigative services. Beyond this, even the choice of medications and the duration of follow-up can vary significantly between different health care providers. Some practices and hospitals discharge patients the same day after a procedure, and others will keep the same patient admitted overnight, or in some cases for a few days. AI can help us sift through data linked to a multitude of such practices and help prioritize value over variance.

DECIPHERING EMR SECRETS

Automated methods using machine learning to risk-stratify, predict, prioritize, and prevent minor or major turbulences in the clinical course of a disease are what we need. As alluded to earlier, there are differing needs for data for different patients at different stages of their ailments. Data could be used just for monitoring the chronicity and stability of the illness, preventing progression and exacerbations of gouty arthritis, dementia, neurological disorders, cancer recurrences, heart failure, and nonhealing wounds. Much of this can be done remotely but is dependent on the right kind of data in the right amount with the right flow. Despite the growing need, there remains an overall lack of a collective strategy on managing and dealing with this data. More than four-fifths of the data in EMRs are in the form of unstructured notes from clinicians. And much of the secret to personalized care lies here.

The approach to analyzing this is far different from the one used for structured data. This is where deep learning and the use of new data science methods, such as natural language processing to extract the content from the clinical notes into a structured format, come into play. The principal underlying thesis to providing high-value care is centered around being able to predict disease or clinical trajectories, so we can provide personalized care to intervene at the right time and place. This could be a simple medication adjustment, modification of a habit seen to affect the course of the disease, or something as complex as an invasive procedure to mitigate the progression or cure the illness. It is here that the use of machine learning and natural language processing can facilitate the extraction of information from the EMR, and this, coupled with continuous streaming data from sensors, could provide the appropriate direction. Whether the focus is on cancer, heart disease, mental illness, or dementia, the strategy remains the same. Much of this will become possible through AI-assisted transcriptions of clinician-patient interactions in a way that we can then use the information most efficiently in an unbiased way.

The practice of medicine is evolving at a steadfast pace. One can envisage technician-aided remote-monitoring services that examine trends and patterns and flag clinically meaningful events for several thousand patients at a time. Fast-forward, and much of this pattern recognition will be run by AI algorithms with some clinician oversight. Some of the individualized decisions that would be hastened and translated into improved clinical outcomes using clinical decision analysis tools to address simple directed questions integrating data from sensors and devices include the timing of starting a blood thinner drug in patients vulnerable to strokes, diuretics in a heart failure patient, or the administration of steroids to a patient with an asthma flare. As patients get older and have many coexisting disease conditions, each one interacts with the others, and these decision-analysis tools become more complicated and convoluted.

Complex conditions such as cancer, kidney failure, Parkinson's disease, or multiple sclerosis are always challenging, especially while trying to use sensor data to predict a readmission event or sudden flare in the Parkinson's or multiple sclerosis patient. We know that false alarms can drive distrust of the patient and clinicians, and costs through the delivery of unnecessary care. This highlights the importance of data that is integrated from multiple sensors with the right intelligence. The hope is that in the future we will have closed-loop systems, where the sensed signal will generate an autonomous response, all within a self-contained loop. Many sensors can generate data, but these are singular metrics, and their adoption across the board into daily clinical care will hinge upon the integration with workflow. There is no simple way to integrate all the information and data from multiple different sensors, especially as there continues to be an endless evolution of the data sources. Very simplistically, a health data platform will integrate information from the EMR, a network gateway for approved medical devices, and a host of evolving sources of data—environmental, social, genetic, biosensors, wearables, and so on. The data from all these sources, before becoming subject to machine learning and algorithm development, require a mechanism for storage, annotation, curation, and aggregation.

The practice of personalized medicine involves the use of every possible data point, whether it be genetics, lifestyle, environmental, or social information in addition to the conventional disease variables that exist in the EMR. Machine learning can dissect health and genomic data and recognize patterns formerly unrecognized by researchers. This not only enables assessment of baseline risk but, importantly, can tell us in real time what the probability of developing a certain condition or disease may be. If we have baseline continuous data on an individual, real-time perturbations can be quickly captured, interpreted, and intervened upon. This could help predict and prevent disease. Collating and analyzing all this free-flowing data is humanly impossible. Machines can change that.

WILL DOCTORS GET LAZY AND STUPID?

Gone are the days of reading voluminous medical textbooks, memorizing innumerable pieces of information, imbibing details of diseases, then regurgitating them on demand. I still get a sense of anxiety as I remember my medical school days, pacing up and down in my hostel room, trying my level best to fill my unwilling cerebral cortex with all kinds of factoids and trivia that would probably never be asked of me in real-life practice. All under the presumption that the mind cannot see what it does not know—hence knowing as much as I could was important. Knowledge was power; it helped differentiate the real Gods of Medicine from the lesser humans.

But times have changed, with all the medical students and residents on attending rounds on the inpatient service stand wielding their smartphones. You ask a clinical question, and everyone's thumbs begin to work to see who can get to the answer first. Quicker, but certainly not smarter. Maybe extracting the right information from the encyclopedia within the smartphone is the new definition of intelligence—or laziness? Whether this change in the use of information technology, coupled with a greater adoption of virtual care, will change the phenotype of medical school applicants in the future remains to be seen.

There is a natural predisposition for us to get progressively more and more dependent on technology, case in point being our smartphones. When there is a widespread belief that the technology could be a whole lot smarter than you, it's easier not to do the hard work of thinking and taking responsibility for some tough decisions. There is someone or something else to blame. We all look over our shoulders to see how we need to act in unfamiliar situations. This is based on observing the actions of others, what could be called "social affirmation." Some of this will change to AI-affirmation, as AI-based advice becomes the point of reference. AI may acquire a reputation of superior standing to social affirmation on the premise that it has constant and seamless access to information across the World Wide Web. Recent experiments have shown that we all trust AI. In fact, many consider it the ultimate truth. Reliance on AI can stifle the use of one's own cortical synapses to solve problems. This creates a dependency. This is exactly how there is an increased dependency of human operators on automated systems, to the extent that it may even dull our ability to troubleshoot. Also, errors generated by faulty algorithms may become increasingly challenging to detect and confront. The bottom line is that it is important for us to construct standards on the use of AI, especially in the setting of critical life-and-death decisions. The *A* in *AI* may be defined as *artificial*, but it needs to be more assistive than automated.

There are some other downstream negative impacts. Paradoxical as this may sound, I think we need to be prepared for this: as we cut back on the need to do repetitive tasks, our energies may be redirected to engaging at higher levels of intentional and intellectual efforts. It is unclear whether this would really save labor, as oftentimes the intellectual tasks are more tiring, certainly emotionally. It looks like such a progression could cut both ways. Also, if the system becomes more efficient, then the throughput automatically increases. It is quite possible that the consequent increase in volume would result in less time for personal interactions and shared decision-making. On the pretext of efficiency and cost cutting, and in the name of personalized medicine, AI could end up being burdensome and negatively affect the patient-clinician relationship. Some of this might even be at the expense of the core elements of empathy and compassion. Maybe AI can make us dependent, blunt our clinical acumen, and bleed our intellect—but most likely it will not allow us to become lazy.

CONTINUOUS INTELLIGENCE—THE REAL THING!

Isn't intelligence continuous? Are we not constantly thinking, analyzing, and taking action? Even the simple act of typing or not typing on a laptop is a form of continuous intelligence. Similarly, just making breakfast, then sitting down and eating it with a complex array of utensils is a form of continuous intelligence. Every second, our heart is beating and pumping blood through all our organs, which in turn, in their own way, are continuously intelligently operative. On that note, does it not seem realistic to be able to uninterruptedly evaluate the functionality of the entire human body on a beat-to-beat basis? This is where the analogy of the automobile or airplane becomes relevant again. It makes sense to have an organ-specific or whole-body digital dashboard being updated nonstop to guide us as we stray from a state of well-being.

In fact, one of the most innovative aspects of AI that may change the landscape of health care is the ability to incorporate continuous intelligence into our day-to-day decisions. The incessant data streaming in from the IoT coupled with cloud-enabled increased scalability allow for the infrastructure that could promote continuous intelligence. Scientists have predicted that, in the near future, continuous intelligence will be mainstream and used more consistently to improve real-time decision-making. Any temporary out-of-range swing in a variable could be picked up on a beat-to-beat basis and accordingly alert the physician to intervene. It could be a single- or integrated-measure alert, depending on what is being measured and for what clinical condition.

A single variable, such as blood glucose or blood pressure, transmitted by a wearable device could alert both the patient and the physician. The continuous-intelligence component, if appropriately trained, will also be able to automatically provide a solution or an intervention strategy to the patient and the physician, using the prior assimilated knowledge about the patient. In complex diseases, such as cancer or neurological, lung, or cardiovascular conditions, the use of multiple wearable biosensors with on-the-spot testing from analytes could help provide streaming intelligence on the clinical course of the patient. And then we have edge computing, which moves network management away from the centralized cloud and toward more localized devices, making everything work smoother, smarter, and with reduced response times. This could help devices become network antennae maintaining Wi-Fi communication between billions of users and devices. The power of 6G could enable collaborative AI within these sensors, medical devices, wearables, phones, and widgets, to better predict, prevent, and treat disease.

Continuous intelligence is also useful within the health care setting to enhance operational efficiencies, fiscal viability, and sustainability, especially if external market forces and the social environment are constantly changing and require the system to keep adapting. Trusting AI, and especially continuous intelligence, will require getting familiar with the underlying logic. Acceptance of AI is eventually going to depend on how much of it is explainable and how much of the black box we can unravel. Adoption of continuous intelligence will be based on trust . . . and within that lies the future of care.

SOLVING BIAS: CAN AI HELP?

I could be treating a seventy-five-year-old white, a thirty-year-old brown, a forty-seven-year-old Asian, or a fifty-five-year-old Black man or woman with hypertension, and my treatment strategy would be essentially the same. If the baseline blood pressures were comparable, most clinicians would start with the same dose of a diuretic or a vasodilator. Crazy, right? What may surprise you is that the clinical trials that make these recommendations were primarily conducted in a white population. Even though we know that there are racial and ethnic variances in metabolism and pharmacokinetics, there is no clear data to guide care in communities of color. Everything is extrapolated. And this does not even take into consideration the host of other clinical covariates, environmental, and social factors that may be distinctly different between these communities.

Medical AI has a data-diversity conundrum that needs to be recognized. Besides the race element, the proportion of women in these studies is so exceedingly small that one has to overlook this widespread bias and hope that the physiology matches up. Most clinical trials have an inherent bias. This is a big problem. This is the whopping drawback of current machine-learning algorithms being generated from large datasets that are noninclusive and thereby nonrepresentative. Whether these are algorithms for risk predictions, disease diagnosis, or treatment, they can be flawed and limited in their widespread applicability.

As a case in point, researchers in Heidelberg, Germany, perfected an algorithm to identify melanoma. They used deep learning to evaluate more than one hundred thousand photographs of skin lesions that were prelabeled as malignant or benign to help the computer reverse-engineer an algorithm. Guess what? The algorithm worked better than certified dermatologists to make the correct diagnosis. The bigger issue was that the algorithm was trained primarily on white skin. The generalizability of this algorithm to diagnose melanoma correctly in other skin colors or tones was marginal at best. This exemplifies that algorithms, like the people who created them, can be biased. Bias can also be created by missing data. Several machine-learning research papers published in prestigious journals have derived algorithms by imputing data to fill gaps. This may further the bias, especially if the data already was not diverse enough.

Garbage in leads to garbage out. If the quality of data is poor or corrupted, the resulting output is going to be useless. Similarly, if the data streaming was collected with bias, the product is going to have bias and be imperfect in its generalizability across the population. Bias can find its way into AI at multiple stages. It can be in the data collection, the classification of the outcome, and the type of technology being used. If the data collected is insufficient, then algorithms generated will not be representative of the problem at hand. Depending on the extent of inclusiveness, the solution may not account for age, race, body mass index, gender, income, zip code, or socioeconomic status. Such algorithms or solutions may worsen the divide and enhance the disparities.

Importantly, these biases often are inherent, not intentional, and so the preparatory segment of defining the intent of the study and extent of the data gathering is the most important phase. Sometimes AI algorithms may be designed for specific locations, regions, or populations. In that case it becomes important to make sure they remain confined to that population and carefully evaluated before generalizing them more widely. At a time when the world is struggling with systemic bias and racism, we need technology that can alleviate health disparities, not further them.

BIAS AND HARM

Biased models have issues. They can result in injury, death, or sometimes increase the intensity of the illness. They can adversely affect the operations of a laboratory or industry, resulting in loss of time and money. The algorithm is usually a black box, and it can take a while before the inconsistency of results points in the direction of some inherent bias. Many are already skeptical of the role of AI, and all it takes is a solitary bad experience to erode trust in the field of AI. There is no systematic approach to eliminate bias yet, and eliminating bias is dependent on the integrity and precision of the researchers in this space. Data scientists need to accept that bias exists, identify the gaps, figure out best practices, and work through the ethics.

There is this ongoing race to be the first to publish and the first to market. Consequently, the need for speed often compromises thoroughness, and among the first elements to be overlooked are personal prejudices and bias. The most important place to examine bias is within the creation of the datasets that we use. Second is to ensure that the outcomes are categorized and adjudicated uniformly and preferably prospectively. If one is looking at large datasets or registries, it is important to ascertain that they are not primarily comprised of white Caucasians of European ancestry, which is usually the case, but that there is adequate heterogeneity and representation from other communities of color and descent. A homogeneous dataset will enhance the statistical power to have a quick working algorithm but will compromise the generalizability; however, if the intent is to develop a race- and gender-specific algorithm, that needs to be stated up front.

UNDERSTANDING BIAS AND FIXING IT

Bias begets bias. Bias goes beyond the dataset to the developers of the AI tool and the contributing role of the lack of diversity in the framers of the question and the founders of the AI algorithm. Depending on the dataset being merged, especially if they are large registries or those from clinical trials, we know quite well that women and minorities are significantly underrepresented. It is key to recognize this and correct the imbalance as we drift into the world of data streaming in from wearables. The data coming in will be much larger, and consequently, so will the bias. It has been well said by video game developer Zoë Quinn that "algorithms are not arbiters of objective truth and fairness simply because they're math."

Treating bias within an algorithm is not easy. If the algorithm does not work, it is easier to change one's expectations than to revisit the whole algorithm. The lack of insight into the way decisions are being made by a machine-learning algorithm is one of the biggest limitations of quickly addressing the issue. Prying open and dissecting these black boxes for their inherent bias or errors is not easy. Sometimes the results can be biased by the way the AI tool interprets the data. An algorithm distinguishing an airplane from a car may be doing so by examining the background of the sky and that of the road, simply because most pictures of planes are in the sky, and those of cars are on the road. It is important to know how the algorithm is reaching its conclusion. The same is important in the interpretation of signals coming from wearable sensors. Missing data and adherence can create bias. AI algorithms used in clinical care need to be evaluated with the same rigor as a new drug or intervention. Every upgrade or modification of the algorithm must be subjected to a similar level of scrutiny. There needs to be a systematized approach that is scalable and deployable, as AI-based diagnostic strategies and therapeutics are going to keep increasing exponentially.

Bias is often an issue of perspective. It depends on whether one is looking from the inside out or the outside in. It can result from who is collecting the data, how it is being examined, and by whom. Medicine is a multiorgan team sport with multiple stakeholders with different vantage points. The use of multidisciplinary teams of clinicians, researchers, data scientists, epidemiologists, and pharmacists is a way to limit this bias. Beyond this, the industry is itself vested in eliminating bias as much as possible. Microsoft and IBM are working on creating automated bias-detector algorithms. Google recently released a What-If Tool, which is an open-source algorithm that assesses the fairness of machine-learning models. It is easier to fix bias in datasets than in people, and that may be the way of using AI to level the playing field in the delivery of care among humans of different races, genders, and socioeconomic status.

13

PREDICTING AND PREVENTING DEATH

If the rate of change on the outside exceeds the rate of change on the inside, the end is near.
JACK WELCH

Maya was a thirty-eight-year-old postdoctoral fellow working in a start-up that was exploring cutting-edge immune-based therapies. She was a mother of seven-year-old twins and married to a friend of mine. She was a spirited young lady with a zest for life, loved her kids, was very successful professionally, and was on a rapid trajectory toward prominent leadership within her company. She was one of the few people I knew who could do it all and make it look easy. In June 2018, I got a call from her husband, asking me whether I could connect him with a specific cancer specialist at my hospital. His voice was quivering with emotion as he told me that Maya had just been diagnosed with pancreatic cancer.

Earlier that week Maya had suddenly developed severe abdominal pain radiating to her back. It was intense enough that she had to go to the ER. The working diagnosis was a gallbladder stone. The ultrasound was inconclusive, and an MRI showed a large mass in the head of the pancreas with metastatic lesions in her liver and spine—hence the pain. Here was a beautiful, dynamic young mother, with no prior medical history of any concern, no family history of cancer, or any recognizable risk factors, who had just received a death sentence. The odds were a 95 percent chance of death in the next six months. Maya, eternal optimist that she was, decided to fight the disease with all her might, hoping that she would make the cut for the lucky 5 percent.

My wife is an oncologist, and through her circle of influence, we were able to get Maya an appointment with the specialist within the next few hours. The following week she was on chemotherapy. The tumor was inoperable, and the hope was that the chemotherapy would help shrink it, which might then allow for surgery to become an option. Maya died four months later.

Our inability to predict and prevent similar situations across a spectrum of illnesses that are occurring around us every second of the day reflects our ignorance of much beyond what the mind already knows and the eye clearly sees. We need machines to complement our intellect, and the big question is whether we can make that happen. Will the advent of the EMR world help provide these answers? Unfortunately, much of what we do today is Band-Aid after Band-Aid. The hospital system thrives on a piecemeal approach to the role of the EMR, primarily using it as a billing tool without a clear holistic vision to predict the unknown. We need to figure out a mechanism to develop, test, and scale technologies and predictive models within the bureaucracy of a hospital environment, which is so heavily sub-stratified into silos and specialties.

Whether one is trying to create integrated strategies to predict and prevent cardiovascular diseases, advance regenerative medicine, create immune- and nanoparticle-based drug-delivery systems to fight cancer, stave off communicable diseases, cure connective tissue or metabolic diseases, or develop innovative imaging modalities to identify subtle changes that may forecast an ominous clinical outcome, we need to work together. There are many problems to solve here, and refined AI approaches seem like they have descended upon us at the right time.

The lightning speed with which evidence becomes outdated after it is published is unbelievable. The COVID experience has shown this to us in real time. Every day there has been an update that disproves a therapy or a theory that was considered mainstream just a week prior. This is best exemplified by the hydroxychloroquine treatment that was strongly advocated at the onset of the pandemic and quickly found to have untoward effects, and may have even increased deaths due to cardiac side effects. I personally received the infamous hydroxychloroquine-azithromycin combination myself when I was ill with COVID. Fast-forward to two months later, and it was no longer on the pharmacy of any hospital in the United States. Trying to keep pace with these changing data and making decisions too quickly during times of duress and stress or trying to calculate probability in a fluid situation is fraught with conceivable oversights. Again, AI-derived logic and algorithms may help us make sense of this information overflow.

RECATEGORIZING DISEASE

We need to revisit disease definitions, risk stratification, and treatments as AI continues to show us the evidence within the body of the iceberg below the surface. Present-day treatments driven by artificial categories may soon change as AI reclassifies and categorizes disease conditions. This will cause us to rethink the taxonomy of common clinical conditions that we may erroneously think we comprehend very well.

I use heart failure as an example again because this is a resource-intensive clinical condition, and solutions to this complex condition can be extrapolated to most other disease states. Now we know (as I noted in an earlier section) that when heart failure progresses, it can cause multiorgan failure. One of the biggest fears in patients with heart failure is that they are prone to life-threatening rhythm disturbances and sudden death. The best time-tested risk-stratification tool to predict this has been the left ventricular ejection (a measure of heart function). Many studies have shown that a low ejection fraction (of less than 35 percent) ferrets out the vulnerable population who may benefit from having a defibrillator device implanted in their chest to counteract a life-threatening arrhythmia by shocking the heart back into a normal rhythm. Now, this may seem rather simplistic, because the human body is so complex; using just one variable (i.e., heart function) to classify someone as high risk seems rather silly.

Well, it probably is, because we have found that, over time, we have been implanting too many of these devices in our patients—several hundred thousand and growing. For every twenty devices implanted, only one may save a life. Although the doctors' intentions have been good, many patients who have the devices implanted in their chest never need to use them. More distressing is that a significant proportion of patients who do not get the device actually succumb to a malignant rhythm disturbance. Many of us have tried to perfect this risk model by adding other clinical covariates such as age, gender, kidney function, and severity of preexisting coronary artery disease to enrich the population who may most benefit from this therapy. Predictably, these derived regression models or risk scores have been incapable of providing enough value to become a part of the patient selection process. They may increase the specificity, but they clearly miss the bus on sensitivity. A part of this is due to the uncertainties of interactions with many other clinical factors that may not be accounted for within the model. To add to this, we know there is a spectrum of social, environmental, economic, and ethnic factors that may amplify this risk, none of which are involved in our decision-making. Just to give you an idea, the cost of each of these defibrillator devices varies widely depending on the type of device, the vendor, the hospital contract, and the region of the country they are being implanted in. It is a multibillion-dollar industry, seeking to be perfected.

In the setting of this costly imperfection, there have been attempts to use AI to better risk-stratify this cohort of patients. A recent study from Sweden using machine learning examined a population of more than forty thousand patients with heart failure and was able to cluster the patients into four different groups. They found interactions between many variables that recategorized patients into different risk groups, very different from the conventional simplistic breakdown based on heart function. It so happened that the Swedish study showed a cluster of patients with a low heart function with certain accompanying clinical traits that did very well, while there were those with a normal heart function who were at high risk of dying suddenly. This exemplifies the point that maybe we need to revisit our categorization of heart failure and taxonomy of the disease, and reevaluate all the evidence that has accrued to date.

As computational capacity within the hospital system expands, machine learning for risk prediction will increase. This will obviously use larger databases inclusive of proteomics, genomics, and environmental and lifestyle influences. EMRs held on central servers will allow for the development of new algorithms via cloud computing, thereby enabling the use of the algorithm in the appropriate clinical environment via the appropriate application program interface (API). Amid the cacophony of algorithms, deep learning, and neural networks, the real challenge for us will be in distinguishing aspirational dreams from reality. But hopefully, within these boundaries, we will be able to ensnare diseases like what thirty-eight-year-old Maya suffered, even before they have a molecular presence, so we can prevent, if not cure, them. The progress will be iterative and incremental. There will be much pain before we begin to see any form of gain. Things will get a whole lot more complex before they begin to get simpler.

CAN WE PREVENT SUDDEN DEATH, HEART FAILURE, AND HEART ATTACKS?

I met Alex for the first time in the ER on a Sunday afternoon. This was twenty-two years ago, when he was forty-two years old and I was a trainee in cardiology. Alex had arrived at the ER with a massive heart attack. He described intolerable discomfort, akin to an elephant sitting on his chest. He complained of a constricting feeling in his chest accompanied by difficulty breathing. This had prompted him to call 911. By the time the EMTs got to him, he was writhing in pain, cold, clammy, and very close to passing out. The EMTs recorded an ECG in the field that showed Alex was in the throes of an expanding myocardial infarction. The ECG showed active and acute injury of the front wall of the heart. We rushed him to the cardiac catheterization laboratory, where we found that the major coronary artery (the left anterior descending artery) was completely occluded. It is often called a widow-maker lesion, and it almost did just that.

Following the diagnosis, we threaded another catheter up into the coronary artery to dissolve the clot and found a severe residual narrowing of the main blood vessel in the heart. The narrowing in the coronary artery was ballooned and dilated, then kept pried apart with a stent left in place. This managed to help reestablish blood flow to the threatened portion of the heart. His chest pain disappeared, and he was stabilized and moved to the coronary care unit, where he stayed overnight. Alex was discharged from the hospital three days later with a relatively preserved heart function. They say time is muscle, and the timely intervention saved his heart muscle from damage. More than two decades later, Alex continues to do well and remains my patient. As much as he won't admit it, he lives in fear of having another heart attack and not knowing whether he will make it this time.

Alex did not have any conventional risk factors for heart disease. He was a young, athletic man of Greek heritage with no vices. His intake of alcohol was limited to social consumption once or twice a week in complete moderation.

He did not smoke or have any of the other risk factors that we know, namely, diabetes, hypertension, or high cholesterol. He saw his primary care doctor on an annual basis and had a normal ECG about four years prior and, in line with established practice, never had it repeated. He was a small-business owner who owned and operated a couple of restaurants with his wife and brother and, in his own words, claimed to lead a stress-free life. He always thought things seemed pretty much in control. I could not explain to him why he developed a heart attack and hypothesized that he may have had a small cholesterol plaque in his coronary artery that ruptured or had a coronary spasm. It was totally unclear. This remains one of the big ordeals of practicing modern medicine, that it all does not always fit. As in Maya's case, many things beyond conventional knowledge don't fit into the spectrum of our understanding of disease and outcomes.

Even though cardiovascular disease (CVD) is one of the leading causes of morbidity and mortality, the contemporary approaches to diagnosis, care, and treatment are rather simplistic. We still predict the future risk of cardiovascular disease based on well-established risk factors such as hypertension, cholesterol, age, smoking, and diabetes. And that's pretty much all we understand at this stage. Our understanding of genetics is improving, but it is still in its infancy. And we know that no one gene will be responsible, but that an interplay of several genes, combined with social and environmental factors, may be the culprit. So, like Alex, there remains a large population of patients at risk despite not having any of the conventional risk factors. On the flip side, there are others who, despite having several risk factors, never have a heart attack.

More than half of heart attacks and strokes occur in individuals who may never have been predicted to have one using conventional risk-scoring systems. We often think that risk factors have a linear relationship to cardiovascular disease, and the worse your risk profile, the higher the likelihood of heart disease. This is true, but only in part. The relationship between disease and risk features is more nuanced. It is here that machine learning, using Big Data, deciphers and teases out the complexity of those nonlinear interactions between a variety of habits, social, environmental, and clinical risk factors and aids in narrowing the gap of our understanding between predicted and observed outcomes. It may not be possible to decode and untangle the explanation of the association, but it will certainly open our eyes to a number of possibilities that may exist beyond our current understanding of human physiology. We tend to use what we have, and that means using risk scores derived from cohorts of patients from the West to make predictions in patients from the East. We know this does not work well. There is more to measuring risk, beyond the conventional risk factors that we know to unmeasured covariates that are more population specific. This has been further substantiated by research from Southeast Asia showing that population-specific machine-learning algorithms are markedly superior to the conventional Western risk scores for predicting mortality after heart attacks.

When one thinks of preventing cardiovascular disease (or any disease, for that matter), prevention can be put into play at three different levels. This could be at the primordial level, which involves the prevention of even the development of risk factors, or at the primary level, which is geared toward preventing the onset of cardiovascular disease in those who already have cardiovascular risk factors. The third level is secondary prevention, which is geared toward preventing disease progression in patients with established cardiovascular disease. The guiding principles for the integration of sensors and AI in risk prediction and preventing disease in these patients remains the same.

RISK PREDICTION: A MOVING TARGET

Who would have ever thought that you could look at an ECG and predict what the heart function is and what it can be in the future? It almost seems implausible that a summated electrical signal (via an ECG) recorded from the surface of the chest wall can tell us about the structure and function of the heart. Not only that, but it can also predict what the heart may look like in twenty years. A simple twelve-lead ECG can forecast which of us may have a heart attack, develop atrial fibrillation, or die suddenly in the years to come. Scary, yet so incredibly powerful!

These insights from a simple ECG are now possible through deep learning. After researchers trained an algorithm to recognize these outcomes from scanning millions of ECGs, the AI algorithm can read minor changes in the electrical signals that are not perceptible or meaningful to the human eye. But if a simple ECG can give us that information, it could assist clinicians to put preventative practices into play and also convince patients to become more compliant to the recommended lifestyle changes. It is possible that if the PCP knew from Alex's routine ECG four years prior to his heart attack that he was at risk, maybe the course of events could have been different.

Beyond risk prediction, trained deep-learning algorithms can now accurately classify ambulatory ECG data. In fact, this works better than the average cardiologist. A recent study that examined the analysis from a deep neural network compared to a committee consensus showed that AI does statistically better with a greater level of reproducibility. As mentioned before, some of our recent efforts have been to use machine learning to automatically measure critical ECG intervals, such as the QT interval, to predict risk for life-threatening arrhythmias. Not just that, but we have begun to do this on a single simple strip of electrical signals from a smartwatch. This could be a game changer on risk prediction and care delivery in so many ways.

Beyond the ECG, AI has been also deployed to assess and read echocardiograms. The difference is that an echocardiogram is a two-dimensional image that actively demonstrates a moving (contracting) heart. This means breaking the algorithm into many phases and then integrating them. AI can now help quantify the ejection fraction of the heart with a high level of accuracy. The manual method of measuring this is a laborious process that involves manually annotating the endocardium, which is the inner lining of the heart, in different views during both the contraction and relaxation phase. This is again subject to manual systematic and random errors. AI can significantly improve the accuracy, reproducibility, and efficiency of the entire process. It will require walking many miles before we can run with this dynamic form of AI.

Further refinement has enabled AI to move beyond the computing function to understand the disease itself. AI can now diagnose amyloid heart disease (deposits of amyloid fibrils in the heart) and hypertrophic cardiomyopathy (an abnormal thickening of the heart). Developing these algorithms requires the use of several thousand echocardiograms to help develop and test the algorithm. There has been a recent move from the conventional large echocardiography machines to point-of-care, smartphone-based assessment via the use of handheld echo machines. Add machine learning to this, and you can totally understand how there will be not only reduced variance in practice but greater global access to technology and expert level of care.

Whether it is the cardiac ICU or surgical ICU, AI is the future of acute care. There is so much happening so fast in the ICU that even though one may be an experienced clinician or intensivist, a lot can be missed. Researchers are using telemonitoring and hemodynamic data in the ICU setting to predict which patient may begin to suddenly slide in the wrong direction. The prediction algorithms will become more robust as the dataset they are based on gets bigger and more sophisticated. Even hemodynamic support systems for the failing heart (e.g., Impella Heart Pump) or critically ill patients are now connecting to cloud-based remote-monitoring platforms. These systems are now able to predict the next six minutes of arterial pressure patterns and forecast a patient's collapse, giving clinicians lead time to prevent it from happening. And then there are AI systems that can screen the entire inpatient population in the ICU, and even the entire hospital, for sepsis, enabling rapid and focused care.

DISRUPTION ACROSS DIVERSE DISEASE STATES

AI has fascinating implications for how the care of patients will look in many arenas. An area that has always intrigued scientists is technologies that can meld the human mind with machines. Brain-computer interfaces (BCI), once relegated to the world of sci-fi, are now real-world entities. Although these may still be in their infancy, they hold promise in the treatment of devastating neurological ailments often associated with paralysis. It is conceivable for people with paralysis to regain their power. Patients with either quadriplegia or a condition known as locked-in syndrome once again can communicate with their families and loved ones. BCIs are propelled by AI-enabled high-level computer algorithms that can rapidly decode the complex electrical activity traversing the cerebral cortex. They can translate this information into digital action, such as typing on a keyboard, moving a robotic limb, or interpreting visual images. Researchers combining AI with BCI have helped patients with paralysis regain the sense of touch, which is critical to any activity. This also allows patients to initiate mobility through "thinking" for tasks such as picking up a fork or a glass. The introduction of electrodes into the brain in an area that processes touch, coupled with sensors in the hand, creates a connection that allows the patient to feel again. These are investigational at this point, but there is promise that AI-enhanced neurotechnology will be able to restore power and sensation and facilitate communication in patients distraught by paralysis. An integration of sensors and AI technology has created prosthetic limbs with built-in video cameras that give a sense of objects' sizes and shapes, potentially getting patients back some normalcy in their lives. This would not be possible without integrated intelligence. Using deep-learning techniques, the computer clarifies the objects and then uses its functions to pinch, pick up, or grasp.

Managing strokes has already been improved using telestroke services, where neurologists at remote sites can help guide care for patients in community hospitals or in rural settings. One of the impediments is being able to both image patients and interpret the results quickly so that therapy can be instituted. Recent FDA clearance of neuroimaging for stroke care was a much-awaited shot in the arm. This enables the pinpointing of areas in the brain susceptible to sustained, irreversible injury that may be eligible for urgent thrombectomy. This can allow a faster triage and transfer to tertiary hospitals, enhancing outcomes. Although the software for Rapid AI was built from more than 650,000 scans from across the world, these algorithms are only as good as the dataset from which they were created.

As discussed previously, type 1 diabetic patients do not produce insulin and hence require the daily administration of insulin via a pump or multiple injections. There is a constant need for dose adjustments, and regrettably in the real-world environment, a patient might wait for several weeks before getting an appointment with an endocrinologist to get to the right insulin dose. Hence the need for an AI algorithm that can help patients better self-manage on a day-to-day, even hourly, basis. A recent AI algorithm developed by scientists enables continuous insulin-dose adjustments for diabetics, working from sensor-aided glucose monitoring.

In the field of ophthalmology, the use of AI to diagnose diabetic retinopathy and other retinal diseases has already found a firm footing. Another exciting use of AI is in trying to cure blindness. The human retina has limited capability for regeneration, and so the progressive loss of neurons can result in complete loss of vision. AI, through the use of conventional neural networks, can help in the recognition and differentiation of stem cells into retinal cells. This has brought us a step closer to the development of cellular therapy for retinal diseases. As mobile processors get smaller, it is possible that AI will support each of the sensor functions, be it vision, hearing, touch, or cognition. As an example of this, a sophisticated form of integration of multiple sensors with AI is "walking like a human." This could involve integration of computer vision and natural language processing to help a blind person navigate. AI-facilitated visual cues that sighted people have while walking along paths, steps, curbs, corners, roads, intersections, and sidewalks could be continuously delivered to the visually impaired along with sensor feedback helping individuals get from place to place.

What about Maya's case? Again, when it comes to cancer, there is so much that goes under the radar. We know that cancers can occur as the result of an interplay of several factors, such as an unexplained intrinsic susceptibility, a genetic predisposition, an environmental trigger or carcinogenic agent, an immunity issue, a spontaneous mutation, or something that we have still not thought of or can't quantify. After Maya's death, I am not sure any of the oncologists were any smarter about how to have predicted or prevented this. Deep learning, using large numbers of scans in patients who go on to develop pancreatic cancer in the future, may provide us some predictive insight. Machine learning with large clinical datasets of previously unmeasured environmental and social factors may help shine some light. An organ dashboard with continuous monitoring via sensor strategies may proactively pick up an early "blip" in pancreatic function. Will this be timely enough to predict and prevent pancreatic cancer, or at least improve the odds toward a higher cure rate? Time will tell. But clearly, there is much work to be done!

14

FIXES, FAILURES, AND THE FUTURE

We must accept finite disappointment, but never lose infinite hope.
MARTIN LUTHER KING JR.

Can AI be our holy grail? Can it fix all health care ills, increase the value of care, and improve diagnosis, risk prediction, and treatment while decreasing physician burden and improving the patient experience?

There are many echelons within which AI can be phased into current clinical practice. These can be cataloged depending on the level and area of disruption, that is, on the extent of impact it will have on the autonomy of the clinician and practice. Although the level of disruption may seem low when using AI at the backend to help with patient flow, the impact on efficiency can be quite significant—for example, by processing vast amounts of enterprise-wide information to organize the flow of thousands of patients through the hospital system, triaging patients from the ER to appropriate locations of the hospital after acknowledging the acuity and relevant bed availability, or helping with patient flow in an ambulatory setting. Using AI in this role seems quite palatable to most clinicians. It allows them to stay in control while undiscernibly enhancing workflow and efficiency. When AI is directed toward assisting the clinician with the decision-making process and changing the workflow, however, it impinges upon physician autonomy and may be looked upon as a threat—especially by a cadre of clinicians who have been set in their ways for years.

FIXING BED CAPACITY

One of the biggest issues in modern-day practice is bed capacity. I can't tell you how difficult it is trying to accommodate transfers into a hospital with no open beds. It is groundhog day every day. The emergency room is diverting patients to other hospitals (often to the competition) because there are no open beds. Patients get held in the emergency room for several hours, and on occasion for more than twenty-four hours, as there is nowhere to put them. Patient care and experience are at their nadir in these situations. Often, elective admissions or procedures get canceled because there are no vacant beds to put them in. This is a country-wide phenomenon in tertiary-care centers that has been going on for years.

Hospitals have several administrators on the case, where there are morning and late-evening bed-capacity meetings; there is a team of nurses and doctors working to help triage patients as their full-time job. They help doctors and teams on hospital floors make decisions regarding discharges and shift patients from ICUs to the regular floors to make room for emergency transfers. Crazy, eh? What a tremendous waste of resources and intellect. Using AI for bed-traffic control and patient placement seems like a no-brainer. As soon as a patient enters the hospital, a machine-learning algorithm screens the current and planned bed-occupancy data. The patient's clinical profile, acuity, infective status, and organ affliction—along with a horde of other clinical features—are processed by the computer algorithm. The AI analytical tool compares the data extracted with a previously developed optimization model built from several thousand patient encounters over several months.

Using machine-learning approaches, the AI helps assign the patient to one of the predefined clusters from the testing and validation datasets used in the past. This analysis is based on successes and failures from the preceding months. This then enables the most appropriate allotment of the bed and shrinks the triage period by severalfold while improving the accuracy of bed placement in the right region of the hospital, augmenting outcomes. Revisiting the influence of bias here is important, as local biases can influence care pathways. And algorithms may be hospital specific and not generalizable across other institutions.

PATIENT FLOW AND UPSTREAM EFFICIENCY

In the outpatient arena there are many places that AI could and will affect care. AI has found a significant role in the backend of office operations, improving flow, creating efficiencies in filling appointment slots proactively in a systematized manner, or taking care of last-minute cancellations and filling them speedily and automatically. Beyond this, virtual assistant tools are finding their way into arming patients with information prior to their clinic visit. I think we have all at some time gone to Google or another search engine to ensure the symptoms we are experiencing are not life-threatening or those of some long-term illness. I have had many patients google their palpitations or chest pain and call me in a state of high anxiety thinking they are having a heart attack or fearing they may suddenly drop dead.

Despite reassurances, they often end up going to the emergency room, as it is challenging to assuage their fears over a phone call. Many times, patients use the World Wide Web to establish a diagnosis before they even see their doctor. Online symptom checkers have been shown to help with establishing a diagnosis and answering questions. This usually involves typing in one's symptoms and answering a few questions. Now there are new apps, tools, and virtual assistants designed to do exactly this, automatically. Isabel is a diagnostic support system that, using natural language processing, can quickly probe a database of more than ten thousand conditions. There are many such symptom checkers, but the big problem is that they all suffer from an accuracy rate of less than 50 percent. This can have many negative downstream consequences, especially if the diagnosis is off the mark.

For outpatient virtual visits or online interactions, machine-learning algorithms can help identify clinical issues, establish a diagnosis, and even suggest a treatment. This usually involves the patient first interfacing with the smart software that asks many questions, integrates the information, and presents it to the clinician to help cut clinic visit time. This is conveyed to the provider, who approves the treatment suggested. Post-approval, the AI system can send the remote diagnosis and prescriptions to the patient. More than 75 percent of this virtual patient interaction can occur via AI. Such AI-heavy encounters are already finding their way into a first-line defense strategy for the treatment of skin problems, wound healing, and hypertension. It is not clear yet whether this will be the right form of communication for all patients, but it certainly could serve the Gen Zs who are looking for a quick solution. When it comes to quick, how quick is too quick? Bright.md is an example of a smart exam platform that could potentially reduce a patient visit time from fifteen minutes to two minutes, thereby allowing an increase in patient volume from 30 to 150 a day. As stated earlier, this upstream positive efficiency could have downstream negative impacts on clinician lives. The fast flow and rapid turnover will diminish the time spent in personal interaction, and thereby the human touch. The possibility of care becoming overtly transactional is a looming threat.

What about the ER? Can AI help there? There is already analytical AI software that allows for continuous ER flow monitoring. They are far from perfect at this stage but provide alerts and reminders to the staff when the wait time of a patient crosses the alert threshold. Also, algorithms overseeing bed capacity and distribution data hasten the identification of impediments and bottlenecks before they even occur. There is evidence that the implementation of such approaches can reduce wait times from arrival to getting to a hospital inpatient bed by 20 percent. One can imagine that as these algorithms get more sophisticated and keep learning in an unsupervised or supervised way, they will be able to make the system progressively more efficient.

The effectiveness of AI within a practice can be manifold and is determined by the lens with which it is viewed. Anything that can reduce redundancy and the burnout of multiple clicks and unnecessary paperwork seems like a natural value-add step. Hospitals and insurers are developing algorithms that can determine the eligibility of a patient for admission, testing, or procedures. Much of this can be assessed in an automated fashion, thereby obviating the need for the back-and-forth of pre-authorizations required in contemporary practice. AI does seem more effective if it is behind the scenes in scheduling and expediting appointments. Its success depends on its scalability and integration with the health care system and EMR.

OPPORTUNITIES AND DISTRACTIONS

AI and its ability to parse through Big Data can provide value at many levels. A simple way to look at this is through its role in risk stratification and prevention. As a reminder, this can be a fairly dynamic process and a moving target within a patient or a particular disease. In the practice of medicine, prevention comes in many forms.

As stated earlier, primary prevention is determining the risk for a group of healthy individuals of developing a particular disease—for example, ulcerative colitis, sarcoidosis, kidney failure, epilepsy, stroke, cancer, or liver cirrhosis. Using the EMR and/or genomic information, the AI-data team could help predict and thereby prevent these diseases. This is primary prevention. And then there are patients with a disease who are at risk of an exacerbation or worsening. This is where secondary prevention plays a role in preventing patients from an acute relapse, deterioration, or hospitalization. Here, AI-directed strategies in patients with chronic diseases can help direct patients on pathways to better health. AI may also help with the tertiary prevention of complications or disabilities of a particular condition. A simple example of the latter on a large scale is the use of passive sensors and AI to prevent falls in the elderly and the frail, who may or may not have other illnesses. Considering the shifting demographics and the rising proportion of senior citizens, one can recognize the value of this if deployed at a population level.

They say the bigger the problem, the bigger the opportunity. More than a trillion dollars are wasted on an annual basis because of the lack of information sharing across institutions. Lack of interoperability and the absence of standardization of data is a big problem. Another important fact that we consistently overlook is that the data guiding care derived from a clinical trial population may not be reflective of the patient we are caring for. That's just a real-world variance (from curated populations for the study) and brings into question our practice protocols. Will guidelines still exist if we can measure patient-directed outcomes in a more individualized way, using algorithms derived from large real-world populations? Most guidelines are directed at the "median patient." They reflect averaged strategies that are anything but precision medicine. Do we then change the taxonomy of the disease, abandon randomized clinical trials, and truly individualize care? It is quite probable that this will be the case, but are we able to trust the AI-assisted decisions? Especially if the AI-suggested intervention or diagnosis may move beyond the ability of the human mind or the physician brain to clearly explain the rationale. Will this black-box phenomena hamper adoption and force us to revisit old assumptions?

So how do we deal with this black-box effect? Most importantly, having confidence in the data quality, its curation, and relevance to the population to which the algorithm is being applied. As an example, with the advent of new therapies and treatment protocols, imaging, and diagnostic modalities, the same algorithm would need to be revisited and refined, as it would no longer be relevant. The workings of the algorithm need to be transparent to engender faith. As data comes in and advances continue to be absorbed into practice, the algorithms need to be adaptive and flexible. Locked algorithms will not stand the test of time.

Deconstructing this black box has also been aided by innovation. For example, within the field of radiology, there are ongoing attempts to increase doctors' ability to understand the plausibility of the results of an AI analysis. Using breast imaging as a model, a pixel-to-pixel logic generates a heat map that shows a direct relationship to the visual information the conventional radiologist can see. This correlation between the AI read and the manual read spawns faith in the AI logic, making the adoption easier. Also, there are heat maps that are now being generated within datasets to show how closely the individual being evaluated clinically correlates with the population from which the algorithm was derived. This gives confidence in the potential relevance of the AI-derived analytics.

Clinical assessment of algorithms via randomized trials will remain challenging. It is well understood that algorithms are not perfect and have to be allowed to continue to learn. But when is that learning enough to lock it and use in a clinical trial? In datasets used to derive the algorithms, were the therapies used optimized and sufficiently standardized? Was the data diverse enough? Computer scientists and clinical trialists are going to struggle with how to assess the utility of a software algorithm as a medical device or drug equivalent while hoping it is safe and adaptable.

Whether we can innovate ourselves out of the cost conundrum into fiscal sustainability is the trillion-dollar question. AI for drug discovery, treatment approaches, improving outcomes, and enabling the focusing of care on the sickest patients in the in-hospital environment show promise. Much of this will be dependent on stepping out of silos, sharing data, and changing workflows while empowering the patient to be a discerning customer who can help us make smarter decisions. Companies are investing at every level of AI, from patient data and risk analytics to medical imaging and diagnostics, lifestyle management and monitoring, nutrition, wearables, inpatient and hospital management, ERs, and so on. There is a projected savings from AI algorithm implementation of more than $150 billion by 2026 in the areas of robot-assisted care, virtual nursing, administrative workflow, fraud detection, dosage-error reduction, clinical trials, automatic image diagnosis, and cybersecurity. (I discuss this in detail in Chapter 18.)

AUTOMATING SURGERY?

In the past I have used magnetic navigation using Stereotaxis equipment to perform procedures. I could sit out in the console room, more than twelve feet from the patient, and maneuver the catheters within the heart using joysticks. The equipment enhances the precision of catheter movement and targets specific areas within the heart that could be causing the rhythm disturbance, while reducing my exposure to fluoroscopy. The natural next step is the use of AI to automatically navigate the catheter to the region of interest and, after some confirmatory tests, deliver the heat energy to destroy the circuit and terminate the arrhythmia. We have already begun using holographic augmented reality technology (SentiAR) to get a real-time, interactive, three-dimensional reflection of the anatomy of the inner surface of the heart. Holographic images with automatic navigation of the catheters may sound fictional, but in reality, we're almost there.

The intersection of AI with interventional and surgical specialties is going to raise a multitude of ethical issues. Most of these relate to bias and accountability. The ethical issues will get magnified as we drift into a completely autonomous mode of operations. This is of particular importance in AI-initiated responses or interventions that would be self-directed. As discussed at length in another section, the datasets used to train AI can be biased to start with. This will create ethical challenges, especially if the downstream impact is dissimilar in diverse patient subgroups. This could mean different interventions leading to different outcomes in different patients.

Let's use cosmetic surgery as an illustration. AI can now predict an individual's age by recognizing facial features that may have contributed to that evaluation. This in turn helps to suggest surgical procedural steps that could reduce the age by modifying those features. Cosmetic surgery is a big thing in South Korea. Surgeons use motion-sensor surgical instruments that collect data in real time and guide the surgeon to make micro-adjustments to improve the outcome. But these AI algorithms have some inherent biases. In 2013, the

Miss Korea pageant created a stir because of the similarity in facial features among those contestants who'd had cosmetic surgery. Beauty, they say, is in the beholder's eye, and this gets even more complicated if that eye is being dictated by an artificial intelligence. It goes without saying that AI algorithms such as this will not be generalizable across a variety of communities and ethnicities.

In a surgical environment or in a procedural laboratory, there is a lot more at stake. An AI-trained robot either freezing because of a technical issue or going out of control during the procedure while dissecting, suturing, or manipulating catheters inside the heart can lead to a catastrophic outcome. The ethical issues will be directly proportional to the extent of AI engagement. When training robots, it would be important to train them with datasets of thousands of procedures performed in a variety of conditions at different sites with multiple operators. Avoiding harm is going to be key. And when that does occur, who is responsible? Will it be the company that developed the autonomously operating robot, the surgeon, the hospital, or the contributors to the dataset?

AI cannot replicate the decisions surgeons make based on gut instinct. The gut-guidance reflex is tough to encapsulate and replace, as much of it is gained from unquantifiable clinical experience. Also, a single complete surgical operation requires thousands of intricate steps, involving cutting, dissecting, excising, connecting, burning, cooling, clamping, ligating, and suturing. For the foreseeable future, robots will serve only to assist; as they become more facile with basic functions, additional layers of complexity will be added, but ever so carefully.

FIGHTING THIS PANDEMIC AND THE NEXT

COVID-19 continues to ravage America and the world as I write this, posing a huge health care, psychological, and economic challenge to the well-being of our society. The pandemic certainly set our innovation engines in motion, specifically to prevent the spread of the virus, but also importantly, to become ready for any resurgence in the coming years. We have already seen many variants and recurrent surges. The pandemic showed us the need to examine large datasets as they come in from across the world with extensive computing capabilities to study the patterns of spread and provide insights toward next steps.

AI has a big role here, not only in predicting spread but in speeding up research and treatment. In the post-pandemic world, artificial intelligence approaches to support remote care and empower sensor-aided self-management strategies will play an important role in defraying cost, reallocating resources, and managing future natural disasters and catastrophic events that threaten human life.

In the fight against COVID, AI has allowed for scalable and adaptive countermeasures on several fronts. Computational advances that include patient information, socioeconomic data, zip codes, and other data with the use of machine-learning algorithms have provided insights toward directing treatment efforts and advancing outcomes across a wide range of locations and clinical presentations. In response to the COVID-19 pandemic, machine-learning-enabled chatbots have emerged to help patients navigate their care. Chatbots, using conversant AI, improved the patient experience while helping screen patients for symptoms. They also assisted in triaging and the provision of educational resources to patients. All this happens without contact. These chatbots, or virtual assistants such as the Amazon Alexa, have access to updated information and can answer the millions of questions coming in about symptoms and care pathways. Even call center responses could be AI assisted. Natural language processing helps perform a sentiment analysis, then using voice analysis can quantify distress and age of the caller, among other variables, to help prioritize the response.

Understanding the spread of COVID-19 has remained a challenge, and AI seems to be finding a role here. Early in the pandemic, BlueDot, a Canadian start-up using AI for detecting disease outbreaks, was able to initiate the alarm regarding the outbreak in Wuhan, China. The machine-learning system for BlueDot was able to deal with large amounts of data, whether they came from news reports across the globe, the airline industry, or clinical practices and hospital systems. This provided information to hospitals and public health leadership regarding the spread, anticipation of new hot spots, and direct resources and efforts at quelling the spread. This was important to enable planning for the potential influx of infected patients, availability of hospital beds, capacity of local ERs, and deciding about the duration of mitigation approaches.

Another AI startup, ClosedLoop, using a vulnerability index, was able to target susceptible individuals in high-risk regions and help public health officials to direct resources, supplies, and educational tools to keep them safe.

Cloud-based AI tactics like this allow for the wider dissemination of these models across the country and the globe. It's not only about detecting hot spots but about predicting regions vulnerable to infections and those provinces that may have a high risk of complications from COVID-19. Then it is also about predicting outcomes and developing algorithms to target patients who will become more severely ill. Some of this may involve focusing on risk factors that may contribute to their worsening condition, thereby preventing mild cases from becoming worse. The bottom line, however, is data, and lots of it—all of it annotated, clean, and with clear outcomes.

AI-based monitoring of social forums in real time can also help gauge the severity and spread of public health emergencies. This could be through tracking certain terms within the social media babble, following changes in travel and spending patterns, or piquing curiosity through conversations connected to cases and deaths. Through tracking Reddit conversations, the trends showed that handwashing and masks became more prevalent topics of discussion only a month after the pandemic hit the US. Having social media sites tied to people's thoughts and actions can help ensure tracking and controlling spread. Researchers at Penn Medicine's Center for Digital Health applied machine learning and natural language processing to Reddit forums. Daniel Stokes and colleagues showed that monitoring the shift in conversations could have provided opportunities for interventions early on to prevent the spread of COVID. There are also apps, sensors aided by AI to track health and behavior in high-risk individuals. These are being used to construct algorithms to better understand individual susceptibility, so as to institute measures to protect the vulnerable.

Much of the undulation in the prevalence curves across the US and other countries has been a consequence of the absence of data-driven decision-making. The hold of COVID-19 has been exacerbated by the lack of predictive analytics, or at least a failure to use them to their fullest advantage. Machine-learning models now enable the accurate estimate of transmission. AI models combining history, symptoms, laboratory testing, and imaging can provide an instant diagnosis, even before the results of the PCR testing for COVID become available.

It seems probable that alternative methods using AI with clinical information may be better than testing kits, paving the path for dealing with future pandemics. AI can help us be prepared for the next pandemic in ways beyond just helping with prediction of spread and tracking. Large volumes of datasets available from medical imaging have helped create algorithms to read X-rays and CT scans that can predict the clinical course and triage patients to the appropriate level of acuity. Scientists from New York University developed an AI-derived method to help triage patients from the ER. This had two parts to it. The first part uses deep neural networks to predict prognosis via the chest X-ray; the second component adds power to the X-ray information by using a machine-learning model to help fold in the results of routine laboratory tests. Algorithms inclusive of other clinical parameters and laboratory markers can help further predict the in-hospital course. Although this was specifically used for COVID, the same technology can be replicated across a spectrum of disease states.

There have been concurrent efforts to integrate the use of AI in drug development and even vaccine development. During the COVID pandemic, we have seen how this integration shortened vaccine development by several years. Beyond this, it also allows for screening compounds based on modeling for mutations of variants of the virus that may come to visit us in the future. There are AI companies developing cloud-based approaches and algorithms to risk-stratify, predict, and recommend treatment. Cloud-based technologies will play a role in supply chain decisions and shortages. For example, the use of predictive analytics will help pinpoint where the supply of personal protective equipment is limited and how allocation needs to change. We will be able to better predict resurgences, and so estimate the potential demand and constraints on resources. It will give us lead time to be prepared for the next eventuality. Because without a doubt, there will be one.

PART IV

MAKING OUR SYSTEM SUSTAINABLE

15

THE VALUE PROPOSITION AND INCENTIVIZING CHANGE

Digital transformation is not about technology. It is about redefining the organization value proposition and ultimately redesigning of the organization.

DR. JEANNE ROSS

My pager went off at 6:59 a.m. on a Sunday. You would have thought that I would be used to this loud, high-frequency sound by now. But no! It still wakes me up with a jolt and sends my heart racing. Sunday is my one day of the week that I like to sleep in late, especially when I am not scheduled to be on call. But here I was, rudely awakened by a paging system that should have figured out that I was meant to be unavailable. Extremely annoyed that I had forgotten to sign out my pager, I was now compelled to respond. I picked up the phone and did my best to sound engaged and concerned, despite not feeling so in the least. It was seventy-three-year-old Marcia, whom I had known for almost eleven years and whose sweet, hesitant, apologetic voice instantly melted my heart. I know when someone pages me at 6:59 a.m., that means they have been patiently waiting for the clock to strike a reasonable hour before calling their doctor. I knew instantly that the issue on hand had been playing on her mind for the last several hours and she had done her best to be patient and find the right time to call me. It was a simple question. She had missed her evening dose of her blood thinner, and she was not sure whether to double up the morning dose to compensate for the missed pill or whether she could forgo it.

A very common question with a simple answer. But clearly this was something that had created enough angst that she had to page me on a Sunday morning. Marcia had had a previous stroke, from which she had fortunately recovered. She had suffered complete paralysis of the left side of her body and had now gotten almost back to normal. Coupled with this, she had worsening kidney disease, an abdominal aortic aneurysm, and multiple myeloma (a blood cancer) in remission. She was one of those unlucky ones who had been dealt a bad hand. She was petrified of having another stroke, and she knew her risk for a recurrence was inordinately high.

It is not uncommon for clinicians to get paged at all hours and on weekends to attend urgently to a patient-related concern. Often, these may not even be urgent. To the patient it is a scary situation, which may not seem the same to the doctor. It's about the vantage point. What is of value to the patient may not rate high on the physician's value scale. What is valuable to the physician may count as fluff to the payer. If it does not save money, then it may not count as high value to the health plans that pay hospitals. At that instant, I certainly believed I had provided a valuable service, and so did Marcia. But this was just another clinical encounter with limited impact or standing from the point of generating revenue. It would have been nice if Marcia's anxiety could have been resolved in an expedient manner several hours earlier. It was a simple enough question that could have been addressed by a health care navigator. It did not need a nurse, advanced care practitioner, or doctor to answer. Or maybe a self-management protocol supported by an algorithm addressing such personal queries could have resolved this simple issue, keeping folks on both sides of the phone call content and well served. I could have slept a tad longer, and Marcia would have had no reason for even a moment of anxiety. Several million similar phone calls daily could be avoided by putting into place the right processes and workflows—that could be digitally enabled, algorithm driven, individualized, and supported at the backend by a caring clinician as needed.

THE NEED FOR VALUE

The argument over shifting medicine from volume to value has been going on for more than a decade. This debate is intrinsic to how medicine will need to evolve, so it makes sense to spend some time discussing this. The biggest issue has been that defining value is challenging because of the multiple stakeholders. Even though patients may define value as compassionate, timely care with minimal personal cost, insurance companies define it (rather impersonally) as overall population health at the lowest cost possible. Physicians feel caught in the middle and fear that, in either direction, the pursuit of value-based care will adversely affect their practices and the bottom line. Agreeing on a common value proposition for health care seems to have challenges in store for us.

This requires us to begin thinking out of the box. Whether it may be a visit to the outpatient clinic, urgent care, emergency department, physiotherapy, rehabilitation, inpatient care, or the pharmacy, we need to establish new processes that eliminate the middleman (e.g., insurance companies and referring physicians) and enhance the efficiency of the transaction. The sustainability of such new workflows and ways of treating patients requires change. This change can be at many levels and needs to be supported and driven by data. Data to measure outcomes, influence culture, and incentivize and manage evolving value-based contracts. Investments in technology and building the data infrastructure to enable the use of machine learning will be instrumental in creating future value through personalized care. This would ensure our commitment toward engendering health equity and enabling population-based health initiatives.

It goes without saying that the existing modus operandi and the trajectory of escalating health care costs are untenable. Evidently, much is still lacking within our system in the United States, pertinent to the quality of care we give, the efficiency of its delivery, and the use of available resources. The existing fee-for-service (FFS) models promote incentives for overutilization, increase variance in practice patterns, and compete with innovation. They put self-interest ahead of a collective vision of progress. Clinicians who are incentivized by the volume of patients and the number of clinical interactions are automatically inclined to give more care, some of which may be unnecessary. Standardizing practice patterns around national guidelines, coupled with expectations of care and its quality, can help enhance the value of care.

Specialty services and complex procedures and surgeries that are well reimbursed stand out as "high cost" within the newer payment schemes. In fact, market forces are already beginning to compel subspecialists to redefine the value of what they do on a daily basis, while aiming to gradually cut back on expensive (often high-tech) "low value services." This will significantly affect the revenue stream for subspecialists and also alter their practice patterns, especially as the value of preventative approaches gains more credibility and attention. The intent here is for value to gradually replace volume.

We must remember that value is a moving target, and that its quantification will continue to evolve as "outcomes science" increasingly focuses on clinical outcomes that matter to patients, especially in the realm of digital delivery of care. As stated earlier, a greater adoption of sensors into an automated continuous care model will require us to better understand the change in workflows and technologies to map care and reimbursement. The effort in care delivery will change in amount of time and description, and so will its value, all geared toward better outcomes that are cost effective. In the coming years, there will be an increasing role for the patient in self-management of their diseases, with greater personal financial responsibility toward caring for their illness. This is going to be an important part of the equation to make health care affordable. For example, patients who are noncompliant with their diabetes, cholesterol, or blood pressure medicines could inadvertently increase the burden on their caregivers and the hospital systems as the result of worsening disease, complications, and hospital admissions. In situations like these, patients will either forgo incentives for good wellness practices or face penalties on their personal insurance premium payments.

A step in this direction, where quality and cost containment are made a part of the payment strategy to the caregivers, is the bundled payment approach, implemented many years ago. There is a predetermined dollar amount for clinical care type, be it a disease condition or a procedure. For example, Medicare or private insurance will reimburse a fixed dollar amount for a procedure such as a hip or knee replacement. If the organization is efficient, with good quality of care and outcomes, they will save money, while those organizations whose systems result in prolonged stays and complications will lose money. This is an example where innovation in reimbursement serves to reduce variability in care, enhance transparency, and make clinicians accountable. The endgame here is driven by outcomes, and reduction of practice variance does not equate to a loss of individualized care. Other examples where similar bundling is performed include sepsis, urinary tract infections, coronary artery bypass surgery, acute myocardial infarctions, and heart failure management. Bundling is not easy, but if the life cycle of a disease and a patient are digitally connected through the outpatient, inpatient, and rehabilitation and home-care domains, it could become a lot easier to measure and manage. It becomes an immutable ledger of care that ties the team together.

CREATING VALUE ONLINE

In a recent conversation with a colleague in Delhi, I learned how advanced India is on the technology front. She told me how she was able to schedule online appointments for her mother and coordinate a visit for herself at the same time. No telephone tag, no waiting in long queues, all seamless. She was also able to check in and make payments wirelessly with minimal to no human contact and no conversations with an automated telephone system. In the US, many smaller practices have started to offer online scheduling as they struggle to compete with the large hospital systems. But many of the big tertiary hospitals continue to remain archaic and vested in practice patterns that have been entrenched for decades, in some places for more than a century. The value proposition here is straightforward. It is all about efficiency, accessibility, and an improved patient experience.

Online consultations are becoming more mainstream and are possibly the solution to shortages of medical personnel and inequity of resource distribution. Imagine a physician office devoid of secretaries, where the appointment, consultation, and follow-up scheduling of tests is an entirely digital experience. No waiting on the phone or post-visit telephone tag with physician offices. As enticing as this may sound (or not), altering the conventional patient-physician dynamic is a huge culture change. But the race for this is well on its way. In many small practices and even hospitals in the US and other parts of the world, online scheduling is the norm. At the same time, there are larger premier academic institutions that are not so nimble, that have been discussing this for years but have had their challenges in trying to implement it. To top this off is the old guard, a cohort of senior physicians who are so used to having complete control over their schedules that handing this authority over to the patient is anathema. According to one of my colleagues, this is deriding the sanctity of the patient-physician relationship. Maybe the vulnerability stems from fear of the reversal of the power dynamic.

Online strategies prove to be of value to not just the patient but also the clinician. Clinicians can formally consult each other electronically regarding their patients on simple clinical issues and not have the patient wait several weeks or months to see a specialist. E-consults are gaining considerable traction, especially among teams used to working within the same hospital system. Specific patient-care-related questions can be requested via a peer-to-peer electronic consultation. In our experience at Massachusetts General Hospital, this helps trim down the unnecessary use of specialists for clinical questions that may be straightforward and answered quickly. These can be questions from the primary care physician regarding additional imaging, blood tests, stepping up the dose of a medication, or even an appointment with the specialist. This saves time and resources and results in better, expedient care, thereby providing high value at low costs. The sustainability of cost control for individualized care mandates better integration and incentivization of clinicians.

It is easier to get three specialists on a Zoom call, compared to congregating in person. This is individualized care as a one-stop shop, but without any shopping. My team has recently been doing this with our heart failure patients. We get the nurse practitioner, the cardiologist, the heart failure specialist, and the cardiac electrophysiologist all on the same video call with the patient and the family. Not only is the patient experience quite phenomenal, but the provider experience also is exceptional. We are all together in the same virtual room talking and taking collective responsibility. It doesn't get better than that!

It is common knowledge that most physician practices are beset with cancellations, no-shows, late arrivals, phone calls, refills, and emails. If one were to put a dollar value on the time wasted, it would amount to every doctor losing an equivalent of approximately $5,000 revenue per week. We already know that the no-show or cancellation rate is much lower with telehealth, but this is also the case when patients are able to schedule their own appointments online. The open-table app concept is making inroads into physician practices. This allows patients to access the schedules of their primary or specialty doctors and find a clinic slot that works best for them. And then there are other brave practices that give patients the option of accessing any physician's schedule within the practice, beyond their primary caregiver. This allows patients to switch doctors to suit their schedules. Who would have thought this would be possible? Personal convenience may triumph over continuity of care! This is not necessarily good, but some argue that everything is in the EMR, and that specific-condition-directed care should be feasible.

Digital interactions, a step beyond just scheduling, are certainly more complex. They are not for everybody. A recent study scrutinized more than 1.5 million physician-patient paired consultations from 2008 to 2018, using a range of machine-learning techniques. The aim was to understand patient characteristics and crucial essentials of the interaction that would predict the magnitude of engagement. The results were indisputable; it was more than just one factor that determined the service delivery quality. The consultative dialogue intensity (experience) and physician responsiveness, along with patient characteristics (whether they were established offline patients), were determinants of return visits to the online platform. For millennials and Gen Z and Xers, who spend a substantial amount of their lives on their smartphones, typing rather than talking is more efficient and less stressful; however, the central factor revolves around ensuring patients are happy with the overall experience and willing to return to the online consultation platform. It is more than just the ease of making the appointment.

SHAPING INCENTIVES

The finances of hospital systems and their providers are healthy only if patients are unhealthy. If everyone were well, hospital services would not be needed. Driven often by personal gain, there is a propensity to practice medicine in a way that seeks to promote more care and more expensive care. More imaging and more procedures generate more revenue for the clinician and the hospital. Physicians generating more revenue are looked upon favorably by the administration and suitably rewarded with bonuses. This is where incentives have gone wrong.

Let me explain this with an example of one of my patients, a sixty-two-year-old lawyer seeking consultation with me for recurrent chest pain brought on by moderate levels of exertion. He explains to me that he feels well but gets short of breath with some chest discomfort when he climbs three flights of stairs. This is new. He even finds that he now gets a little winded when he goes for a three-mile run. He is very categorical that this has evolved over the last six months, so not a rapid worsening. He is otherwise feeling fine and can engage in all his day-to-day activities with no limitations whatsoever. There are many ways I can approach this situation. I can spend time understanding his overall situation a little better. I can explore his risk factors, such as high blood pressure and diabetes, and adjust his medications to control his heart rate response with exercise and see how he does. I could institute all these preventative strategies to mitigate his risk factors and potentially help improve his symptoms and thereby prevent a heart attack in the future. On the other hand, I can adjust his medications and arrange for an exercise treadmill test. Or instead, I could consider either a noninvasive imaging of his coronary arteries such as a CT coronary angiogram or lean toward an invasive test such as a cardiac catheterization to examine his coronary arteries. The options are many. They say medicine is an art, and nobody can fault one for choosing any of the above strategies. The choice of strategy is usually dictated by the level of suspicion (a qualitative skill). A variable that subconsciously comes into play here is the relative value unit (RVU) factor (explained later in this chapter). The downstream RVUs and revenue generated, or health care expenses, can vary by several thousand dollars between each of these approaches.

Unfortunately, in many practices and in some regions of the country, such decisions are driven by the potential RVU and revenue it might generate. Using evidence-based medicine, this patient would do quite well to have a conservative approach with risk-factor modification and lifestyle modification. Unfortunately, this does not pay well, while procedures, testing, and imaging do. This is where the current fee-for-service model incentivizes greed. This is where reimbursement models need to change. The system is currently untenable and doomed to failure. Policies that recognize and reward high-quality care while incentivizing outcome-focused decisions over RVU-driven ones are the need of the hour. These will embolden a delivery system positioned on preventative strategies, so we can avert the inexorable amount of spending on pricey procedures that may not be always necessary.

INCENTIVIZING BEHAVIORAL CHANGE

As much as there are fascinating advances in transplants, cell therapies, and minimally invasive procedures, it would be nice to not let disease states progress to such a state that one needs to prescribe expensive medicines, cut skin, and enter the human body to surgically repair a problem. This is where continuous tracking and management of diseases using virtual care with sensors will allow us to treat patients conservatively and help institute timely interventions as and when needed. This is not a Band-Aid approach for treating a symptom, like stenting a narrowed coronary artery until it re-stenoses or waiting until another one gets choked up. Streaming continuous data can help predict and prevent disease while promoting cures. If all risk factors (or at least the ones we recognize at this time) can be kept at bay, one can halt progression and often even regress the severity of the disease. The ultimate goal here is to cure. To exemplify this further, a newly diagnosed type 2 diabetic can be treated with expensive medications, or one could encourage and ensure strict lifestyle modifications that could cure the disease—and I really mean *cure*. It may surprise many, but early forms of diabetes, and sometimes even more advanced ones, are curable.

The success of incentivization lies in fresh models, which will need the existing ones to be completely deconstructed and realigned with newfangled priorities. Incentives will be levied through employers, who pay the premiums for their employees and staff to take ownership of their health. At the clinician level, reimbursement models aided by a "real-time digital register" of care will delineate outcomes and help catalyze the modification of reimbursement models beyond the RVU. Standardization and transparency will be two guiding principles that will help cleanse the system of some of the toxic residues of the current fee-for-all setup.

THE RELATIVE VALUE UNITS SAGA

Maybe the first place to start is understanding how the system is incented. Figuring out the right tactic to incent culture change among clinicians has to come first. Physicians talk in relative value units, also known as RVUs. These are the centerpiece around which the lives of most (but not all) doctors revolve. Every activity engaged in, every patient seen or procedure done, is a mental calculation in RVUs. Time spent away from patient care on a committee or teaching nurses or residents is time spent not generating RVUs. Again, I am generalizing, and sincerely hope I am not undermining the sanctity of the profession by the above statements, but in a way it is still true. Better to work with the truth, if we are thinking of challenging the status quo.

RVUs are almost an obsession. As much as it plays on the doctors' minds constantly, most are repulsed by the fact that their worth is equated to such an inane metric. To further explain this, Medicare uses a fee schedule that elaborates how physicians are paid for more than seventy-five hundred different services across surgical and nonsurgical fields. The fee for each service is valued by RVUs, which have been categorized and ranked on a scale that has been standardized across much of medicine. This rank order is directly dictated by the extent of resources that particular task takes up. This could include physician work, expense of the physician's practice, and liability insurance. It is not entirely clear to most practicing physicians how all this is calculated, but it is quite evident that the task is laborious and also flawed, as it tries to objectively capture the resource requirements across different work environments.

RVUs account for time, technical skill and effort, stress to provide the service, and mental effort and judgment. It is quite evident that many of these supposedly objective criteria are qualitative and subjective. The calculation is further affected by who is on the panel and how the decisions are being made to allocate the RVUs. Also, the RVU remains a moving target, depending on evolving technology, newer procedures, and interventions changing within the specialties. As the skill and effort for any procedure increases, the RVU for that also increases proportionately. For example, the work value for open heart surgery is considerably higher than angioplasty and stenting, although in some cases they may achieve the same result. The same argument could be extrapolated to medical therapy versus interventional approaches. Even though medical therapy in some patients achieves the same result or may even be better, the expense incurred and the RVUs generated are markedly lower. This is how medicine gets weighted more toward procedures or invasive strategies.

It won't surprise you that much of medicine and the health care economy and Wall Street are driven by new, expensive cures, and less by long-term preventative treatments that, in the big scheme of things, may be more meaningful. As we move into an era of digital care that allows for continuous monitoring of patients, enabling earlier remote interventions to prevent disease progression and its downstream consequences, the RVU strategy will need to be revisited. The assessment of the true value of administering care will need to be reassessed. We need to define what is more valuable: the continuous management of patients traversing periods of wellness and sickness to prevent disease, or the expensive, complex downstream interventions that we use to palliate or cure. One approach does not exclude adopting the other when needed. Also, the central immutable feature in life is that there will be a consistent need for wellness. To ensure this, compensation schemes will *need* to change, and the business model will *have* to evolve.

DIGITAL VALUE UNITS: A CONCEPT OF THE FUTURE?

In line with the above argument, there has been a near fiftyfold increase in telemedicine in the US post-COVID, along with doubling of patient interactions, messages, and alerts in patient portals. The accruing distress from the challenge of trying to respond to each message is palpable in the many conversations I've had with primary care physicians. In one such chat with David, a close friend and colleague, I learned that a primary care physician receives on average 350–400 new electronic messages per month via the patient gateway. These are "new" encounters and don't account for the additional back-and-forth that each message can potentially generate. David went on to say that most of this work of responding to messages and emails happens late in the evening (eating into personal time), after most of the other clinical tasks of the day are done. None of this work of staying connected with the patient is recognized, valued, or reimbursed. It is a freebie. As stated earlier, the system recognizes RVUs and units of care. It does not have a mechanism to handle the multiple digital-touch encounters that are so critical to everyday practice and lead to better outcomes.

This is complex. How does one convert multiple digital interactions into units of care? Should a fee be levied to the patient and/or the insurance company for every digital interaction? Can you even imagine how complex and administratively laborious this may become for a practice? And then every billable interaction comes with a co-pay. What was considered free of cost will now begin to bleed the pocket. Equity is threatened, since disadvantaged patients will not be able to afford recurring fees or have provisions to participate in recurrent digital interactions. This complexity of care delivery, unit sizing, and value-adjusting to construct digital value units (DVU) will be a nightmare for patients and physicians. The fee-for-service model is unsustainable as it tries to cultivate parity for payment models across different modes of contact and for varied durations of time. This challenge of reimbursement is driving most clinicians back to the in-person mode of clinic visits. Although the technology is here and delivering health care digitally is possible, the payers don't have the right equation—hence the gravitation to the old ways or burnout with the new ways. Some say the viability of a digital strategy in practice is going to be dependent on the business model for health care. Or maybe this could be better stated: the viability and sustainability of the health care industry revolve around developing the right business model for the implementation of digital care.

The status quo is untenable. A fee-for-service model quantifying and qualifying every digital touch seems rather farfetched. A capitated, value-based model seems to be the only plausible solution. We are at a juncture where innovation and experimentation are essential. Academic medical centers that have their own health plans may be able to help us out of this conundrum. It is about accurately defining the value proposition and incentivizing change to make it happen.

16

CHOOSING THE RIGHT PATH

There is no single right answer or path forward,
but there is one right way to frame the problem.
CLAYTON CHRISTENSEN

It is an honor to have known Harvard Business School Professor Clayton Christensen. Each time I met him, I was struck by his sincerity, humility, and pure genius. If you've never had the opportunity to attend his lectures or watch his videos, his earnest, nonjudgmental, intellectual tone and ability to state things as simply as possible always leave you longing for more. His book *The Innovator's Dilemma* changed the way the business world thinks about disruption and innovation. Taking a page out of his teachings, I think we have an opportunity to use technology to disrupt the structure of the current non-viable health care system. It is not so much about the technology but what we build around it to enable it. Christensen indirectly suggested that swiftly advancing (digital) technology by itself has no way of affecting the world until it is embedded in a successful business model. We are fortunate to exist at a time when there is a real prospect of bringing about this change. We need to better define for our patients what health care can and should look like, rather than conforming to existing needs. And then make it happen!

PATTERNS OF CHANGE

The health care sector is morphing as I write this. The arrival of several known digital companies (e.g., Amazon, Google, Apple, and Samsung) into this space coupled with their all-pervading cloud services have begun to dominate the shape of this evolving landscape. Their nimbleness, customer-friendly strategies, and superior market research will continue to keep them several steps ahead of most hospital systems. Even large health care companies (e.g., Philips and GE) that were slow-moving ships with challenges in this space have begun acquiring start-ups to keep up with primarily digital companies. The focus is now patient-centric. How patients receive care, where they want it, and when they want it will determine the way they get it. Moreover, this will be quite different from patient to patient and disease to disease. Gone are the days of the patients being subservient to the patriarchal medical system. The roles have reversed. It boils down to what an excellent patient experience looks and feels like. A good experience has been shown to lead to better adherence to advice and medications, which in turn leads to better outcomes and cost savings.

The digital industry has been identifying the gaps for several years and trying to plug them with innovations. Apple, for example, was among the first to recognize the far-reaching impact of simple wearables on securing and analyzing health data via the Apple watch. Having found an obvious role in measuring physical activity and assessing heart rate and rhythms, it has even entered the world of clinical trials facilitated by using apps. It is constantly engineering new sensors, apps, and care pathways that could fit into the consumer market in a clinically desirable and potentially durable location. There is also a slew of start-up digital companies, along with the aforementioned giants, that are reshaping the way patients and providers connect with each other. This could start as a transactional connection that is virtual and periodic but morph into a seamless, continuous transmission of digital data (during periods of wellness) that is managed by AI-driven logic. Rather than waiting for patients to fall sick, the care pathways are programmed to predict and prevent.

Professor Christensen has pointed out that in a typical hospital, overhead accounts for nearly 90 percent of total costs, primarily because it is a one-size-fits-none option. There are multiple business models within the same hospital that are mostly incompatible. Combating this overpricing of care requires an unrelenting pursuit of cost-effectiveness. Much of this quest is through enhancing efficiency, but at the expense of investing in innovation. The goal is to combat declining reimbursements by increasing volume. Same care, but delivered more efficiently. In speeding up the delivery of care, the effort has always been to ensure that the quality of care and patient experience are not compromised.

For example, procedures that used to take many days in planning and lengthy stays in the hospital are now outpatient procedures or discharges on the same day of the intervention. Three-week stays for post-heart-attack patients thirty years ago are now two- to three-day admissions. Lengthy surgical procedures are now significantly less invasive with shorter stays. Patients in the past routinely stayed for up to fourteen days after cardiac bypass surgery but now are homeward bound in four. Most orthopedic and urology procedures are now same-day ones. A lot has already changed, but this is only the beginning. Early discharges mean more care at home and a greater reliance on patients managing themselves (with the appropriate guidance). Regardless of where the care is delivered, one can be sure that a sizable segment of the care will be outside the four walls of the hospital. Personal accountability will be a part of the economic equation, either through lifestyle changes, monitoring one's personal sensor data, adjusting doses, or adherence to medications.

SHIFTING CARE COSTS

The financing of health care is likely to change. Right now, as we understand it, health care insurance companies are our payers, and they receive a premium payment from patients that may be disbursed directly by the individual, employers, independent organizations, or government agencies. Health plans classically pool the health risks among all their members and work under the assumption that the larger number of healthy, low-cost members will offset the expenses from the few higher-cost individuals within the plan. The culture of care is moving from making health care all about treating sickness to making it about keeping patients healthy. The hope is that this shift in ideology, with the accompanying changing care patterns focusing on wellness and lifestyle, will in the long run reduce the cost of care.

Much of this kind of care will be virtual. The increase in virtual care will reduce infrastructure needs related to space and staffing and thereby costs. This will also shift the expenditures of providing clinical care. Virtual or video visits are outside the hospital environment, and so the likelihood of using ancillary diagnostic services decreases. Will these savings result in profits for hospitals, or will the parallel decrease in reimbursement have financial implications at the provider level? This will certainly bring down health care costs overall, and the redistribution of these savings will enable the dissemination of more equitable and uniform care. Much of this will be determined by the level of engagement of the payers, insurers, regulators, and Congress, along with hospitals, pharma, and device and tech companies and their lobbyists.

The new economies of an asset-light hospital environment delivering outpatient care outside of the hospital will provide an opportunity to restructure how outpatient practice should look, and how personnel and space should be redistributed. There is always a cascade effect, and with the advent of virtual care and sensors, the care of a subset of inpatients may get shifted to an ambulatory setting. This may adversely affect the level of reimbursement to the hospital and clinicians but, again, will reduce overall health care costs.

This shifting of inpatients to the outpatient arena can be illustrated with the example of the large proportion of patients with atrial fibrillation who are routinely admitted for monitoring during the initiation of a medication to control heart rhythm. This is done in the hospital because the medication can alter the electrical signals in the heart and, instead of controlling the arrhythmia, may result in a life-threatening arrhythmia (ventricular fibrillation) and lead to cardiac arrest and sudden death. Starting this medication in the hospital enables us to record ECGs before and after the initiation of medication and helps mitigate any risk from a predilection to developing an abnormal prolongation of the electrical signal that makes patients vulnerable to sudden death. Though the risk of sudden death is low (about 1–2 percent), it is serious enough that current practice mandates being proactive about this with inpatient monitoring. Now that ECGs can be recorded at home through a wearable, such as a watch or via the AliveCor app, it is not unlikely that patients may begin to be monitored at home, thereby shifting inpatient care to the home-care environment. Recent work from an artificial intelligence company (Cardiologs) highlights the ability of a cloud-based algorithm to measure these electrical signals from the ECG generated by a smartwatch. A study I collaborated on with investigators in France involved monitoring eighty-one COVID outpatients with mild symptoms receiving the controversial hydroxychloroquine-azithromycin combination. We used smartwatches to record ECGs and a cloud-based AI algorithm to monitor the electrical signals. Fortunately, none of the patients had any out-of-hospital life-threatening arrhythmias, and our ability to monitor and predict the risk from the watch ECG was comparable to a conventional ECG recorded within the hospital. Core elements for such innovations to see the light of day will involve safety, efficiency, and staff and patient engagement. Measures like this could save the health care system money but negatively affect the finances of the clinician and hospital. The goal is a good one; it just needs the right business model.

EVOLVING CARE EXPECTATIONS

Care is changing, as are expectations. Consider a patient who is very sick with a failing heart who may prefer to seek care from a digital company that could follow the patient every single moment, as opposed to an office or a hospital-based practice that has many competing interests. If affordable, it would be a no-brainer that one would prefer to be looked after by a team of concierge practitioners who care only for such sick patients. It is what they do best. They carefully track patients digitally all day long and intervene proactively if there is any suggestion from the sensor data trends that the clinical course is not on target.

We know these sensors can predict and detect heart failure several days before it clinically manifests. It's just that, because of resource constraints, clinicians currently have not taken it upon themselves to pay attention to that sensor data on a minute-to-minute basis. Moreover, with primary care physicians or cardiologists managing panels of several hundred patients with a wide spectrum of illnesses outside of heart failure, it is challenging for them to pay individualized attention. And even if they do, it may not be in a timely fashion. This demonstrates a deep gap in the care we provide to this brittle group of patients. Similar analogies can be made across a wide variety of chronic diseases, including diabetes, chronic obstructive lung disease, coronary artery disease, a variety of cancers, and a range of neurological diseases such as Parkinson's, epilepsy, and so on. Time is of the essence. Well-timed recognition of disease progression or flare-ups can help prevent complications and as a result flatten the cost curve.

Patient care spanning the hospital, non-hospital-based practices, disease-specific digital care platforms, and home care will require care coordination and a quarterback. Presently the quarterback may be a primary care physician, but in the future, it could well be a health care navigator (a non-MD) or the well-informed, digitally enabled patients themselves. The goal is to provide the best care, keep the patient well, and save money. Over time, patients and consumers will decide how the health care they receive needs to be valued and who they should be seen by. This will be a moving target that the digital economy, its ledgers, and the accompanying transparency will help better display.

WILL THE FUTURE BE PIECEMEAL CARE?

The accessibility of one's own data, guidance by AI-assisted algorithms, 24-7 access to health care navigators, and freedom from the physical constraints of a hospital building are going to change the dynamics of everyday care, along with the economics for the entire health care industry. The greater control that patients will have over their own lives will change the buying and selling of insurance and care. Insurance premiums with individualized package deals for specific disease management platforms will become a reality. Patient experience will be at its core, and the Uberization principle of health care will prevail. Care will be wherever and whenever, and maybe for whatever! Disease management platforms (explained in the next chapter) run either by the giant digitals or digital care start-ups may be directly answerable to patients for their clinical care. It is quite likely that a patient may opt out of conventional group practices to get their long-term care for their heart failure or diabetes through a specific care package from a disease-specific digital provider. This third party may contract directly with the patient outside of conventional insurance. This would be a new beginning for individualized, piecemeal care. Conventional comprehensive insurance coverage in its current form would still exist, with an option to opt out for specific chronic diseases. This might save on premiums, which could be invested in disease-specific digitals. Of course, some health plans may have their own personalized digital-care deals, blended with conventional coverage and self-management obligations.

Leading health systems are looking to the future. Those that are visionaries are taking risks, not willing to press pause waiting for reimbursement to be formalized for virtual care practices. Efforts are underway to redesign the digital care pathway to make it a consumer-centric, frictionless experience. Organizations are reaching out to the digital-space disruptors for partnerships. Those with less bureaucracy and a greater degree of nimbleness are getting traction from big guns such as Amazon, Google, or Microsoft, who are in an equal hurry. This is where redesigning the care pathways is going to be important, rather than just digitizing conventional practice workflows. Systems are chasing the idea of rethinking our current paralyzed patient-physician interactions and facilitating digital care that is customizable and empathetic. The outpatient, inpatient, emergency room, and pharmacy experiences need a futuristic design that can be stitched together to create a seamless patient journey, one that will endure over the coming years.

THE ASSET-LIGHT CULTURE

Let me reminisce a tad. Bookshops, video rentals, and CD stores are like legacy institutions. We are also seeing other brick-and-mortar stores graduating to becoming showrooms with business models entirely dominated by the digital experience. I still feel exceedingly nostalgic when I see a Barnes & Noble and make a point to walk in and spend some time browsing. But I always realize very quickly that although it is the system I long for, it is highly inefficient and greatly uneconomical. I go in to find a book and after much consternation figure out that it's not on the shelves, and I will either have to order it online or come back in two weeks to pick it up. My analog life has transitioned. I am across the threshold. The nostalgia remains, but just on the fringes, and it may not be too long before that, too, disappears.

Businesses such as Uber and Airbnb have eclipsed their competition, and with a significantly reduced infrastructure. Hospitals will transition toward this model, too, the underlying theme being to become asset light. Remote care during the pandemic showed us that this is possible. The big buildings may become smaller and focus on tertiary and quaternary care, as most primary and secondary care will shift to off-site ambulatory-care locations either close to or in the homes of our patients. The patient home will become an outpatient clinic suite, their bed a hospital bed. Virtual care with sensors will contribute to the reduction in infrastructure and of resources such as staff and personnel. Add to this online scheduling, and now we will have a seamless patient-to-clinician connection from home. On the back end, the creation of an automated or administrative-assisted lineup to expedite tests, questions, and preparation for procedures will make this paperless, predictable, expedient, and an all-in-one experience.

When you bring AI and telemedicine together, there is even the potential to make telemedicine a physician-free experience. This is exactly what the Latin American Telemedicine Infarct Network is trying to do. This network, operating through a hub-and-spoke strategy, has transformed the care pathways in Brazil, Colombia, Mexico, Chile, and Argentina. Telemedicine coverage is provided to a population of a hundred million with an emphasis on helping establish diagnoses and preventing unnecessary transfer of patients to hospitals. Other AI-based efforts to predict heart attacks can be influenced by changing climate conditions (more heart attacks occur during extremely cold weather) and use zip codes to help target care to vulnerable regions in an expedited manner. Much of how we deliver care will be repurposing and redeploying existing resources, and this is where deep-learning methods will help the health care system stay fiscally viable.

The Uber-ization of health care is inevitable. This means care at any time and anywhere, across all borders. This will involve an asset-light health care system with a large number of vetted clinicians all over the world, available 24-7 to opine and provide care to patients. This will need translator services and the ability to refer patients to nearby facilities for tests when needed. These visits will be multidisciplinary, involving more than one specialty, and can beam in family members, social workers, and nutritionists as and when required. Maybe the next success story would revolve around an asset-light organization that could run consultative, research, educational, and outpatient care services across the globe. That would also help create uniformity of care in any global crisis, the pandemic being an example. This will most certainly require overcoming several logistical and regulatory hurdles.

DIGITAL HOMEOSTASIS: THE NEED FOR INTEGRATION

The acceleration of telehealth has created a hunger for sensor-based approaches to provide hard data during a virtual visit. To some extent, this simulates a clinical exam and provides comfort to the provider that they are not "winging" the clinical evaluation. Often a patient feels well, but the sensor data may tell a different story—hence the importance of having objective evidence. As discussed in earlier chapters, the availability of even simple sensor approaches such as heart rate, blood pressure, oxygen saturation, and temperature can augment the value of a virtual visit.

We now have a provision for digitizing different organ functions through sensors. More sensors could equate to better care and provide an assessment of the equilibrium between the different physiological processes within the human body, better termed as digital homeostasis. Although the process is experimental, it is apparent that clinical information regarding cardiac, respiratory, neurological, gastrointestinal, and liver function via sensors will soon be available to evaluate from a distance. Integrating this information at each visit will be possible, provided there is a sustainable business model propping it up. As of yet, there is no single digital company, health care company, or hospital practice that brings all this together. Several start-up digital companies are working at breakneck speed to fill the gaps, but these are just the gaps. Digital practice still lacks a holistic vision, primarily due to regulatory hurdles and the challenge of EMR integration.

The integration of these start-ups with the digital giants, health care industry, or hospitals will result in a new ecosystem: a clinical environment that is driven by sensors and backed by predictive analytic tools. It seems implausible that any company can truly influence clinical care without having its technology linked to the electronic medical record. This is true not just for the start-ups but for all the big digitals. Scaling this integration is not going to be easy, especially with the variability in the adoption of EMRs and practices within the thousands of hospitals across the country. And at the other end are thousands of wearables and widgets that provide the needed data. Each one provides different data and in different forms, and the construct of a single integrated platform almost seems like an impossible undertaking. The information streaming from phones, watches, wearable bracelets, rings and necklaces, tattoos, clips on our clothing and shoes, and so forth makes the simple request for a common portal of entry and exit from the EMR a rather tall order. This information can be collated during wellness as well as disease, where each patient will serve as his or her own control, using their baseline evaluation. Alerts triggered at preset levels will notify the practitioner of a perturbation of the digital homeostasis warranting attention. Continuous streaming data being monitored constantly will change the way we practice.

As sensors continue to evolve, the continuous data acquisition needs to reach a high level of accuracy. While false alarms can overwhelm the clinician and result in increased utilization of resources and downstream costs, subpar detection could have damaging clinical consequences and harm patients. Sensors conveying erroneous information about clinical stability when the patient is progressively declining can lead to disastrous consequences and outcomes. It takes one bad experience to put an end to a great ideology of care delivery.

MYOD

Add to this the Manage Your Own Disease (MYOD) concept, and we are in a different world. Imagine patients taking care of themselves—patients guided by their own data, individualized alerts, alert-specific education, and prescriptions already in place to help expedite care. This is already happening and has been tested in small cohorts of patients. As mentioned in Part I, Chapter 3, I helped lead the international LAPTOP-HF study, where we implanted sensors in the heart that could measure the pressure in the left atrium. This study was undertaken with the aim of limiting readmissions and death in patients with heart failure due to clinical deterioration. The sensor that we implanted in the interatrial septum (the partition between the right and left atrium) was connected via a lead to a pacemaker-like device placed just under the skin below the clavicle. The pressure measured in the left atrium, transmitted via the lead to this device, could be read by placing a handheld gizmo over the device. It indicated whether the left atrial pressure was high, normal, or low with actual numbers that could be compared to the patient's left atrial pressure at baseline. This in turn informed us if the patient was doing poorly, when the left atrial pressure rose above the patient's baseline pressure, and indicated whether there was impending heart failure several days before the patient had clinical symptoms. There were three phases in managing these patients. The initial observation phase was several weeks, where we learned about the patient by tracking their left atrial pressures. The second titration phase was a couple of months, where we assessed the patient's response to changes in medication doses and educated the patient. The third was a prescriptive phase, where the patient managed their own heart failure by checking the left atrial pressure and adjusting the dose of the diuretic medicine based on a scale developed during the titration phase. For example, if the left atrial pressure was up by a certain amount, the patient would self-medicate with a pre-prescribed dose of forty milligrams of furosemide that had been assessed in the titration phase. The goal was to empower the patient to manage themselves to prevent an incipient progression of the disease leading to clinical collapse and hospitalization. Even though the use of an invasive implantable monitor may appear complicated, it doesn't seem so in the real world. We now recognize that selected variables from watches and less invasive subcutaneous monitors can provide comparable and useful surrogates for impending heart failure.

A triggered alarm on a connected smartphone directs the patient to self-adjust their medications based on a well-constructed prescriptive algorithm. Extend this to wearables, and the reduction of millions of hospitalizations would have a profound impact on care delivery and sustainability of the health system. There is also recent work showing that the use of smart technology for blood pressure regulation yields results similar to standard-of-care visits. Extrapolate this to several million patients with high blood pressure who have weekly and monthly in-person blood pressure evaluation and titrations of their medications by their physicians, and now imagine the savings of eliminating those transactional care encounters.

As we move into this realm of self-management for chronic diseases, how should the reimbursement model evolve? In the real world, most of these digital companies can provide a wireless infrastructure enabling self-monitoring. We are already checking our physical activity and heart rate. The incentives currently are quite variable and often self-imposed. These could be to lose weight, get more fit, compete with friends and family, and in some cases, may even have been requested by their health care provider. But as we move beyond the wellness phase into disease, the equation changes. Lifestyle modification is one thing, but disease management is another. As an example, type 2 adult-onset diabetes mellitus is a lifestyle disease that we know is curable in a substantial proportion of patients. Medicines help control the blood sugar and mitigate the long-term downstream complications of this condition, but don't cure the disease. They are used to help treat the metabolic disarray from a poor lifestyle. The cure lies in modifying the lifestyle, with tangible evidence that doing so might even obviate the need for medications.

Let's look at the math. We have 1.2 million diabetics in the United States who could benefit from better lifestyle management and potentially not need medicines. Sensor technology (e.g., FreeStyle Libre and Dexcom) can provide continuous feedback to patients, enabling stringent diet regulation and promoting exercise based on the circadian distribution of blood glucose levels. If patients were encouraged and incentivized to help manage their own disease, billions of dollars would be saved on an annual basis from simple lifestyle intervention. Or do we explore the options of disease management platforms, where patients independently contract with a digital company to help them better manage their disease, separate from their contract with the insurance companies? External contracting driven by the inability of the conventional practices and their clinicians to adequately give the personal attention needed by patients who may have curable or preventable disease states.

Smart technology with individualized algorithms advising drug adjustments either directly or through a health care navigator can save several hundreds of millions of dollars, besides improving the patient experience and averting the need for time-consuming, periodic transactional visits. As has been wisely said, self-care is not self-indulgence, but tantamount to self-preservation.

17

FUTURE MODELS OF CARE

The aim of medicine is to prevent disease and prolong life; the ideal of medicine is to eliminate the need of a physician.
WILLIAM JAMES MAYO

When I walked into my clinic office to greet Brittney, I was surprised to see a young, petite woman who looked quite different from what I had imagined. I had been prepping for this clinic visit by familiarizing myself with her medical chart and her medical history. Instead of seeing someone depressed, emaciated, and listless, I was taken aback by her upbeat persona, how well she looked, and how her smile lit up the room. I was seeing Brittney to help protect her from sudden death while she was being evaluated for a multiple-organ transplant.

Brittney is a thirty-nine-year-old mother of two young girls. She was diagnosed with insulin-dependent diabetes at age eleven and had gotten used to self-injecting with insulin. Despite rigorous control of her diabetes, the disease had begun taking its toll on her body and various organ systems over the course of the last four years. She was developing kidney disease and had been put on medications to help slow the progression of kidney failure. About two years ago, her heart function began to worsen. This came as a surprise, because she felt pretty good and was actively teaching her class of first graders without any limitations. And then a year ago, she developed osteomyelitis, a bone infection involving her big toe. For this she had to receive a six-week course of intravenous antibiotics that inadvertently hurt her kidneys further, and she developed full-blown renal failure. She had gone on dialysis six months ago. By this time her heart condition had worsened despite medications, and now she effectively had kidney, heart, and pancreas failure. She was being evaluated for a triple organ transplant. My job was to implant a defibrillator in her heart so that I could protect her from any fatal heart-rhythm disturbance while she went through the next steps of evaluation of her suitability as a candidate for transplantation. This could take several months or years.

The picture gets a little more complicated when you take into consideration other factors. Brittney lives in rural New Hampshire, and for her to get this care meant that she had to travel multiple times a week to Boston, which is a little over a two-hour drive, one way. Even though she got her dialysis at her local hospital, she had to see multiple specialists across the Mass General Brigham system. Her endocrinologist was at Brigham, her kidney and heart doctors were at Mass General, her primary care and dialysis care was local, close to home, and her general cardiologist was at Wentworth-Douglass Hospital in New Hampshire. She was, in effect, getting her care from four locations, six primary subspecialty clinicians, with another twenty doctors involved in her care as she got her tests and evaluation studies performed, over different practices, hospitals, and states.

One can only imagine how complex it can be to coordinate this care across hospitals and doctors working within their own silos. Also, for the patient, just the hassle of traveling, waiting rooms, variable expectations, different practice patterns, and the additional uncertainty of each clinical encounter can make for a miserable experience. But is this problem fixable? Can we make this better?

This is where the concepts of "systemness" and "networkness" come into play. The hospital system is a dynamic, ever-changing, always morphing behemoth. Some of this evolution is happening organically because of the evolving needs of the hour, and some of it is deliberate in anticipation of the needs of tomorrow. The world of clinical care is evolving from an individual, siloed approach to a much larger form of care called systemness, which in turn can lead to a grander form of connectivity, or what could be called networkness. Networkness is an era of openness, where one can seek care anywhere from anyone. There are no borders and no rules, with a change in the social order of the practice of medicine and care delivery to every human being on this planet.

SYSTEMNESS: THE PATH TO CONNECTIVITY

Regardless of whether you're a patient, doctor, nurse, health care worker of any sort, or an administrator working in a clinical facility, you may have encountered the term *systemness*. There is much banter, some hype, and loads of angst whenever the concept of systemness comes up, including a foreboding sense of doom as clinicians talk about the changing times and how systemness will have a negative impact on their autonomy and the way they look after patients.

Simply put, systemness is the creation of a connected care stratagem across a blend of specialty centers, community hospitals, practices, and ambulatory clinics spread across a large geographical footprint. Some of this could be regional only but also may extend across state boundaries into national and international terrain. This often involves a collective cultural change in the mindset of how hospitals, their subsidiaries, and affiliates need to work together by tweaking their clinical practice patterns, the intent being that the practice patterns, workflow, technologies, data sharing, and even deployment of staff across the different components of the system become seamless, allowing the varied constituents to function collectively as one single entity. The goal is to create an optimal patient-centric experience across the entire system while increasing patient access, improving clinical outcomes, and enhancing the overall quality of care—something that could serve Brittney's care well.

Clearly, it is not easy. Systemness requires a level of integration that creates distinct pressure points among the stakeholders. This discomfiture could be at the level of the practicing physicians, advanced practice providers, nurses, technicians, ancillary support, or administrative staff. Enabling the system to function and provide the highest value care at the population level (which is the goal of systemness) requires powerful leadership to underscore the priorities and break down the organizational silos. The perceived loss of autonomy is a big barrier, as is the replacement of one's independence with interdependence.

Some of these changes are more straightforward and less controversial. These more acceptable components to systemness involve implementing operational changes at the backend, streamlining business functions, and encouraging supply chain efficiencies that will have an immediate impact on efficiency gains in cost, quality, and patient access across the system. It is when the system seeks to standardize clinical practice patterns (reducing inter-physician practice variation) to improve care quality that one's autonomy begins to be threatened. Physicians develop and hone their skill sets over decades of practice and are understandably averse to being told to change elements of their practice overnight. Most of us feel that our identity lies in our exclusivity. Physicians and institutions often subscribe to a similar notion, that they are unique and distinctive. From their perspective, their individuality is threatened by the ask for uniformity in their practice patterns. Technology can provide a helping hand here. Digital connectivity with common dashboards and patient-data sharing across all the components of the system can serve as the glue.

Systemness is a continuous process. The health care system is a living organism that is never static, ever adapting and evolving to the changing times and environment. It enables a path to the greater goal of connectedness. Systemness may be the initiating platform, but the goal is connectivity through networkness, which allows one to get care from any caregiver, anywhere within a system, and even beyond systems—anywhere in the country and across the globe.

NETWORKNESS

Digital transformation is a process of social change that reaches into the value system and norms of our society. The need for connectivity is the catalyst for this transformation. The network does not exist by specific rules, as a system does. It doesn't have boundaries. It is not top-down and hierarchical. It is open and permeable. It enables better access to care and allows patients to seek care where they want, without middle managers and free from the conventional constraints and workflows. There is already an expectation of immediate access to information, and there will be the same for the receipt of clinical care. Conventional hospital systems are incapable of providing that. Importantly, networks exist within systems but also can connect outside of them. This parallel universe of networks calls for us to rethink the organizational model. The parallel structure needs to be integrated into a care pathway that is transparent, open, and trustworthy.

This connectivity has created a new cadre of patients willing to connect outside the conventional system. The e-patient is educated, enabled, engaged, and empowered. Patients are connecting with each other through platforms (e.g., PatientsLikeMe.com) where they can learn through the lived experience of patients facing the same disease-specific challenges. We always forget that patients are experts in living with and having the disease. And, in fact, patients are probably our most underused resource.

As patients move into networks, the business models for care will evolve. To what extent these networks will be covered by insurance schemes in the future versus self-pay will relate to the value proposition. Its impact on costs and outcomes will determine its role in the future. It goes without saying that these networks will grow and transcend conventional geographical and political borders. They will need some governance, but that will need to be within a flexible framework that can continue to evolve and adapt to changing needs. Through networkness will come the opportunity for remote dissemination of digital diagnostics and therapeutics that could enable the long-desired, ever-escaping goal of global health equity.

REMOTE CARE PLATFORMS

Remote care is not new. Over the years, it has had many versions. Early on, remote care comprised telephone-based follow-ups, usually administered by nurses and doctors. This was done for patients who were too sick to travel or may have had compliance issues with their medical regimens. In many cases it did not affect outcomes, because the spacing of follow-ups was too far apart, adherence remained a problem, and the contribution of health inequities was underappreciated. More recently this has evolved to monitoring of data extricated from implantables and wearables from beyond the conventional clinical environment.

As mentioned in earlier chapters, my colleagues and I have been involved in remote monitoring of patients with heart disease for nearly two decades. This has been achieved through implanted devices and sensors such as pacemakers with a unidirectional flow of data from patient to clinician, leading to an intervention by the clinician that usually involves an in-person clinic visit or dose adjustment of a medication to mitigate a potential problem. With the availability of a variety of sensors and a range of digital therapeutics, the potential for remotely managing patients across a slew of different disease subsets is enormous. The impact of this making health care delivery sustainable and cost effective is humongous.

As much as this may appear intuitive, it is extraordinarily challenging. It means changing the culture of practice, altering the mindset of physicians rooted in the comfort of the status quo. It means reinventing the art of medicine so it can operate seamlessly over the network. The wheel of the health care industry turns very slowly. It is superconservative. We spend more time looking down at our feet, to ensure that we don't trip over ourselves, than scoping out and implementing long-term approaches. Presumably, trying to predict the future increases a sense of vulnerability and may not engender a collective, cohesive vision. So playing possum seems like an approach many hospital systems continue to subscribe to. It's just that these systems that are directly responsible for the care of patients are not sprightly when it comes to change. Throw in some bureaucracy, add some regulatory hurdles, and pepper this with inertia, and you have paralysis.

On the other hand, the more agile industry health care companies (e.g., GE and Philips) are pushing for change. They have formed partnerships with software companies to enter the arena of remote care. Like other players in the industry, the goal is to provide caregivers—including health care providers, family members, and patients themselves—a platform to look after patients from a distance. There has been a surge in apps in the recent past. These are aimed primarily at shifting care responsibilities and encouraging a greater degree of self-reliance. An example of this includes apps for helping manage patients in the preprocedural, postoperative, and post-discharge periods. These could also include the delivery of rehab services at home.

The apps being developed for an array of conditions across medicine contain video-assisted advice, instruction, and access to an expert around the clock. Companies such as Medtronic, Abbott, Amwell, and Boston Scientific are establishing disease management platforms to enhance connectivity between health care centers and patients through mobile devices. This would potentially allow for remotely tracking patient information, enabling continuous care, and proactive interventions in patients at high risk for hospitalization or untoward events from disease progression. The emphasis here is to ensure that there is a connection overseeing the transition of a patient from the acute hospital setting to a nonacute setting at home. The home setting is gaining more relevance since patients spend more time at home than at the hospital. Managing patients at home using an array of digital tools can keep them healthy and thereby prevent readmission. This will require a high level of coordination, disease monitoring, data analysis, interpretation, and care instructions.

Digital companies (e.g., VitalConnect and Cadence) offering a suite of connected devices to a remote-monitoring platform have continued to push forward. They have taken it upon themselves to help manage and monitor the sickest of the sick patients. Along with this they are trying to inspire the gargantuan health care system to begin considering new reimbursement models in a valiant attempt to change the culture outside their own organizations. This may sound disruptive and defiant, but the hurdles to change continue to plague this transformation.

Hospitals may decide to construct large remote-monitoring platforms with full-time remote-care physicians and nurses. Job descriptions will need to be redefined, coupled with a repurposing and redeploying of clinicians to these larger setups to provide instant care and reduce the need for in-hospital services. The final confluence will vary within hospitals and systems. It will involve an intersection between technology within the hospitals making it into the homes of patients coupled with personal widgets and gadgets that route from the home via an integrated platform into the hospital. The remote-monitoring platform will need to be an open platform that is agnostic to third-party vendors as hospitals evolve to become modular (discussed later in this chapter). Care will be remote, continuous, exception-based, and as needed, through disease management platforms.

CHRONIC DISEASE, CONTINUOUS CARE, AND SELF-MANAGEMENT

There is an old saying: one disease, long life; no disease, short life. This may sound counterintuitive at first, but it makes a lot of sense. Those who know what's wrong with them and take care of themselves tend to live longer compared to those who have a sense of bravado and consider themselves to be always healthy, neglecting early signs of ill health. Acknowledging early deviations and intervening promptly is the mantra of chronic disease care.

As we embrace remote care, we need to prepare ourselves for the inevitable era of sensor-guided continuous care. Constant free-flowing digital data from watches, wearable sensors, and Bluetooth-enabled monitoring devices will alert us if patients begin to stray from good health. Rather than waiting for patients to fall sick, the care pathways will be programmed to be preemptive. This would be most applicable to chronic diseases. There are estimates that by 2030, eighty-three million Americans will have three or more chronic health conditions, up from thirty-one million in 2015. Continuous digital monitoring with alerts triggered by predefined criteria will enable proactive care of patients with diabetes, hypertension, chronic obstructive lung disease, atrial fibrillation, and heart failure, among a host of other conditions. Some of this is already underway and will involve assessing and monitoring patients during periods of wellness. Electrical signals emanating from sensors on a beat-to-beat, minute-to-minute, hour-to-hour, or day-to-day basis, processed with refined machine-learning techniques, can be condensed into meaningful information that enables early detection, allowing for more efficient clinical decision-making.

Stakeholders (payers, providers, and patients) will need to be incented to enable this culture shift in care. Market forces will need to reinforce the value of previously described shared saving strategies. Encounters will become less transactional, with a move to establish a target amount of expenditure for each patient. At this moment, the true impact of virtual care on downstream future costs remains speculative. Costs, as measured by the hospitals and health care corporations, are short-term and yearly, as opposed to real-world estimates of costs over decades at the individual and population level. On the flip side, virtual care via increased access to care could also result in increased costs. There is the possibility that the absence of personal contact could increase dependency on lab testing and imaging needs, leading to over-testing. The hope, however, is that sophisticated sensors, inexpensive smartphone-assisted point-of-care testing, and keeping the population healthy will drive down health care costs.

THE SHIFTING POWER DYNAMIC

The power dynamic between patients and physicians will continue to shift. Patient empowerment and engagement in the care of their personal health is the goal. In day-to-day practice, patients usually present to the clinician when the illness or condition has progressed to a breaking point or to one of extreme discomfiture. It is self-evident that most disease states start off incipiently with no overt clinical symptoms. Much time is lost waiting for symptoms to develop so that the illness becomes identifiable as a well-defined clinical syndrome that allows the doctor to make a diagnosis. Often it is too late, and the disease has progressed to a point at which it becomes irreversible. Data collection by smartphone sensors and wearables allows the pickup of signals early in the subclinical course of the disease. Digital technology from an array of passive or active sensors enables the recognition of a deviation from the norm, encouraging the patient to seek out medical attention or manage their own disease prior to an exacerbation.

Incentivizing patients for self-management of their chronic diseases has begun to factor into reimbursement models and insurance premiums. The argument stands that self-management will not only reduce the number of emergency room visits but also improve long-term outcomes for some conditions. Currently, there are various insurance plans in place to target patient behavior, including ones that lower premiums if the patient joins a gym (Kaiser Permanente). In parallel to reducing premiums to incentivize patients to engage in healthier behaviors, the reimbursement model involving sensor technology will also engage patients with their own care at a lowered cost to both themselves and the health care system. If patients are incentivized to help manage their own disease, billions of dollars would be saved on an annual basis.

This new digital environment will encourage patient participation within the models of care delivery. Patients will work alongside their clinicians. Patients will be able to feed their objective sensor data into app-assisted algorithms and decision trees that might help them to decide when to seek help. This can be toward managing their cholesterol, blood pressure, blood glucose levels, allergies, or psoriasis. How this will fit into the care pathways, workflow, and day-to-day use of wellness parameters continues to evolve at a jet-fueled pace and depends on the fidelity, accuracy, and interoperability of the signals. Continuous care, codriven by the patient, will lead to reinventing the classification of many disease states, redefining the appropriate time to deliver individualized treatment, and shifting the care-delivery paradigm. The power balance between patients and physicians is ready for disruption. Careful validation and generalizability across all patient groups and demographics will need to be gauged. Hospitals, physicians, and administrators must get ready to test these new care platforms and consider experimenting with innovative sustainable reimbursement models for the future.

EXCEPTION-BASED CARE

Care only when needed seems like a reasonable concept; however, care in its current form (virtual or in person), like conventional outpatient care, remains episodic and transactional via a fee-for-service model. This occurs despite us knowing that disease, or even wellness, is a continuous state and flare-ups do not coincide with our periodic, predetermined follow-up clinic visits. In the peri-pandemic period, as we reengineer our clinical practices, we need to craft an economic model that would encourage the delivery of continuous care but not overburden the system. Maybe there is something to learn from the role of remote monitoring of pacemakers, loop recorders, and defibrillators. In the not-so-distant past, patients with implanted devices were evaluated in person every three months. With the advent of continuous wireless remote monitoring of these devices, patients are now seen once a year, unless there is a problem reported through monitoring that mandates an earlier visit. This is tantamount to "exception-based care," where a patient is followed continuously and treated only as needed when indicated by sensor data. If care was considered only for preset digital alerts, can the model of exception-based care used for implanted devices extend to wearables? Of course, the technology, the data accrued, and its continuous interpretation will need to be robust enough to allow this. But it does seem to be the way forward, especially when dealing with chronic diseases.

A large segment of health care consumers is looking for specific, as-needed care. It could be a urinary tract infection, a common cold, a fever, sinusitis, or a range of other problems that are self-managed and need care only if severe—on an as-needed basis. The catch is that they want it immediately, with no wait time. This is a big market of young patients who would be happy to have immediate care in the middle of the night from a practitioner to whom they could provide some basic sensor-driven data related to their vital signs. Having a prior relationship with a primary care physician is not high on their agenda. The system will change because of the needs of this generation of consumers that is flexing the system to adapt to their needs.

DISEASE MANAGEMENT MODELS

Most start-ups have figured out that trying to develop a singular comprehensive care model across many disease subsets does not work that easily. The nuances of each disease and the need for a specific care pathway pose a distinct challenge, hence the move to disease-specific areas. There is a list of clinical conditions where poor outcomes and quality of care are subject to federal penalties. These fines are imposed upon hospital systems for high readmission rates that increase the cost of care. Several of the aforementioned companies are uniquely positioned to help reduce readmissions for heart failure, chronic obstructive lung disease, asthma flares, post-heart attack, community pneumonia, and so on. The goal is to add value to the caregivers in managing these complex conditions, improving the clinical trajectory of the patient and eventually curbing health care expenses. Again, the way this works itself into a reimbursement strategy is fraught with the high level of variability as to how each hospital has its processes and pathways set in place.

For example, at Massachusetts General Hospital, we have a well-oiled internal machine that assists with post-discharge education, helps schedule outpatient follow-up visits within two weeks of discharge, and has an alert system with a rapid-response team to take care of the patient should they get readmitted to the ER. This works well, and we have one of the lowest post–heart attack readmission rates in the country. Even though it works well, it is intermittent, and the touch points with patients are spread out over several weeks. There is still the danger of things falling through the cracks. Patients may get anxious or have some lingering symptoms that need to be addressed before the scheduled follow-up. It is obvious that a digital system with as-needed video visits and continuously flowing sensor data can make this unified, enhance the patient experience, and potentially improve outcomes. This eventually may even reduce the need for staffing or change the type of staff, and may morph into a dedicated in-person remote-monitoring strategy, which in future could be abetted by algorithms, health care navigators, and chatbots. With the use of AI and its downstream algorithms, human contact may be invoked in a setting of some complexity that requires a higher intelligence. The inertia to invest into this concept is pitted against the minimal incremental change that this may provide on a quality measure (i.e., readmissions) where the hospital already does quite well. Eventually, it boils down to the vision for the future, delineating priorities, and repurposing available resources.

Getting patients to take charge of their health and incenting the adaptive behavioral changes seems important. The system can spend tons of cash on treating the downstream complications of obesity and diabetes, but it will never make it right. It will consistently be playing catch-up. Making it right is treating the root cause. For this, empowering and increasing accountability of patients is going to be essential to making health care for all sustainable. Beyond this, data analytics individualized to the patient clinical condition with customized approaches to deliver medications to ensure adherence will play a role. Simple single-disease conditions such as diabetes, high blood pressure, asthma, skin rash, or allergy flare-ups may involve an alert to the patient and delivery of a prescription to the doorstep. The several in-between steps will become like the mystery of operations revolving around Uber, Netflix, or Airbnb, all of which we now take for granted. A cloud-based infrastructure and advanced remote monitoring that will subsequently enhance care using predictive analytics seems the natural evolution of care. The business model will be dictated by cloud services, patient-friendly innovative widgets providing sensor data, and a tech infrastructure that can be scaled.

The question that comes up in all these disease conditions is whether this digital conduit should be integrated into a reimbursement model where patients self-pay separately for this service or have a capitated model that bets on better outcomes and an improvement in quality measures, whereby the technology pays for itself. The shared-savings model seems like the most plausible solution, where the digital company helps the hospitals save money and may then partake in the profits. Hospitals, physicians, health care providers, and administrators must get ready for similar new care models. These are hurtling toward us with a quickening pace that may well overwhelm us. Only those who have had the vision to plan for this transition will be able to keep stride.

GOING MODULAR

Having personally practiced in India, the UK, and the US, I have had the unique opportunity to see that none of the existing health care systems work well. It is time to rethink the hospital and the health care system in anticipation of evolving business models. Tertiary hospitals and large academic centers may need to reinvent themselves. They must move beyond using digital technology purely for enhancing the backend operations and efficiency of the system. The goal is to disrupt the current mode of conduct and then make it self-sustaining. The essential component toward that goal will be in ensuring that sensor-guided virtual care strategies will improve margins and outcomes and create net growth. Some of this may become a little easier by understanding the job at hand and its multiple components.

Let's use the banking industry as an example. We understand that there is more to the banks than just our checking and saving accounts. Their services cater to a range of needs, some of which may include payment transfers, loans, credit cards, asset management, and mortgages, among a multitude of other functions. As much as we may love our bank and the customer service when we visit the offices in the brick building, most of these functionalities are often better served remotely through dedicated independent platforms such as Venmo, LendingTree.com, Kabbage, and Robinhood, among others. These provide some of the same services that Big Bank provides, but quicker, cheaper, easier to navigate, and infinitely more personalized. Banks are also beginning to realize that having an open modular interface with these newer dedicated platforms may help cut costs and retain their customers' loyalty. Having the right partnerships with the right degree of interdependency will be important for striking a fiscally viable proposition. Though there is some loss of control, the endgame is a success if the customer is getting the best possible experience.

Hospitals are a lot more convoluted than the banking industry. Here we deal with personal issues that are far more complex and involved. It is not a wire transfer or cash withdrawal, but instead often a life-and-death situation; however, the overarching objective is the same—namely, customer satisfaction with good outcomes at lower costs. Today, this goal seems more realizable than it did in the past. The advent of sensors, digital connectivity, and AI now provides an opportunity to disrupt the health care experience by simplifying the inherent complexity. One way to do that is to examine the hospital through the lens of modularity. Will the patient be better served by disease management modules? It so happens a multitude of third-party vendors are doing exactly that—enhancing the individual patient experience. Providing patient-centric care, or what we now recognize as precision medicine. This is different from the experiential, more generalized, guideline-directed population medicine approach that we currently practice. This is where hospital systems may benefit from going modular and developing an interdependence outside their four walls.

ACADEMIC MEDICAL CENTERS: THE EVOLUTION

At the same time, established academic medical centers are morphing and trying to redefine themselves. Frustrated by the inertia and resistance to change, many clinicians are leaving conventional hospital practice to begin start-ups that focus on the delivery of personalized primary care and disease management programs. Deep structural changes that depart from conventional care-delivery architecture are falling into place. New technologies and AI assets are being put into place to create new workflows that will hopefully transcend the boundaries of primary and specialty care. In one such model, the academic center of the future will provide tertiary- and quaternary-level care across state and national borders and focus on rare and complex diseases while working with local third-party vendors for primary care.

Andy Ellner is the founder of Firefly Health, a primary care service that is doing exactly that. Andy's premise is that deep structural changes are needed within the hospital system if we are ever going to realize the dream of health care for all. According to him, telehealth via video visits is a good start, but nowhere close to being enough. The primary care system must evolve beyond the doctor. It must empower and equip a nonphysician team that extends to involve patients and their families. The hierarchical structure of current practice needs to be flattened, with team-based decisions that can occur quickly and include newer workflows, that are no longer fee-for-service, not transactional at every encounter, and no longer built on clinic visits. For this to occur there must be a sustainable, financially viable model.

The Medicare Shared Savings Program has shown that this may be possible. We know that participation in shared-savings contracts by physician groups translates into savings and thereby promotes the concept of "value creation."

Some of these third-party primary care services are clinic-based, with a move toward becoming more and more cloud-based. A few of them (98point6, Firefly Health, and Galileo) contract with private payers, and others, such as Heyday and Patina, work with public payers. The ecosystem is changing, and most of these mushrooming newfangled primary care practices are betting on the fact that digital transformation will break national borders and increase global care opportunities. This will stretch the large academic medical centers, which will morph to meet more complex subspecialty needs while shedding primary care and wellness needs. The fact that patients want cheaper, faster care from their primary care physician, without having to interface with a complicated goliath, will only serve to further this transition.

As care evolves beyond looking after the sick and toward caring for people during periods of wellness (to prevent sickness), it may become a question of bandwidth and fiscal viability that begins to set the stage for this modular approach. There are also disease-specific vendors looking to establish disease management platforms and partake in the risk-sharing of patients over the life cycle of certain disease states, be they diabetes, asthma, certain cancer types that are now like chronic diseases, heart failure, and so on. It might make sense to integrate these vendors and platforms into a risk-shared strategy, helping provide more patient-centric care.

Also, what currently may be considered high volume and low value (i.e., wellness) may become a high value soon, as fee-for-service becomes more and more capitated. (*Capitated care* refers to a fixed amount of monies being allocated to the care of a patient, and whatever is saved becomes the revenue that is generated.) Prevention is becoming the name of the game. An example of such an organization is Forward Health, where the emphasis is on long-term health and preventative care. The clinic visits feel very different from those of a hospital practice. There is no waiting area. Patients glide through an automated scale and red-light spectroscopy station that captures their weight and a thermal map of their body, along with vital signs and oxygen saturation. Before they see the doctor, blood is drawn. If deemed necessary and agreed upon, genetic information from collaborations with 23andMe can also be used to enhance the comprehensive preventative plan during the face-to-face or virtual visit. There are 24-7 chat features and provisions for same-day visits or phone appointments.

Companies like Nudj and Omada have made it their mission to treat and prevent chronic conditions such as hypertension, obesity, and behavioral health issues. These and other similar programs have a team of physicians, nurse practitioners, nurses, physician assistants, health coaches, and behavioral health specialists working in partnership to provide in-person and virtual care. It will be challenging to emulate and scale this model within a large tertiary or academic medical center, not because of the lack of political will or talent but because of the exorbitant overhead expenses to run such programs in large hospitals.

BUILDING ON CONVENIENCE

Convenience is a big deal. It's probably the reason pharmacies integrated with convenience stores in the first place—to create a one-stop shop. But the aim now is to move beyond prescriptions into the arena of providing health care. CVS and Walgreens are in the midst of expanding their footprint by engaging in telehealth. CVS recently merged with Teladoc to provide virtual care with a team of virtual-care nurses. Most issues addressed are focused and straightforward, such as colds, ear pain, rashes, or fever. Walgreens and Rite Aid are right behind with their telemedicine kiosks, where patients can have a confidential consultation and point-of-care testing if needed and pick up their medicines on their way out. Younger consumers are more likely to go to a CVS or a Walgreens for health care than a traditional health care organization. It's important to recognize that convenience is relative and our needs are ever-changing, and this will continue to define the path forward. If conventional hospital setups are not able to adapt and make the entire transaction an easy one, patients will seek urgent and primary care elsewhere.

There is a new generation of health care consumers who have no time for complex personal interactions, especially if all they need is a simple prescription for their acne, rash, allergies, reflux, weight issues, hair loss, or erectile dysfunction. They would rather avoid the human contact and would like to take care of this in their spare time at the end of the day or just before going to bed, on the train, or on a lunch break. This need has spurred the launch of consumer telehealth companies such as Hims, Hers, and Ro. They would prefer to pay out of pocket for easy, immediate access to prescriptions that otherwise would result in embarrassingly long conversations and administrative barriers of authorizations before getting approved by the insurance companies for only a marginally lower price. It is not worth the effort. Some younger consumers are also letting go of their primary care physicians, as they would prefer to maintain their privacy by staying out of the EMRs that too many people have access to. This may not be just limited to healthy younger individuals, but even sicker patients would prefer a concierge-equivalent service and personalized care for their complex diseases. The future will be shaped on the insistence of patients seeking instant, affordable, and on-demand care.

The evolution of the hospital system will eventually depend on its sustainability, which is linked to growth and profitability. How the hospital changes will depend on how it fits into this advancing landscape. This may not be one size fits all, as there could be differences based on the demographics served and availability of subspecialty services. Some of this could be shaped depending on the mission—to serve a few high-margin patients or enhance care for the larger population. Simplistically, one can break up the hospital into three streams. The mainstream comprises wellness modules, the midstream includes chronic diseases and disease management modules, and the upper stream comprises the subspecialty and surgical services. The academic medical center or large hospital system could cater to all three but will have to deal with the nimbler competition in the mid- and mainstream arenas. Going it alone or developing a symbiotic and fruitful interdependence with modular intermediaries will be the billion-dollar question. It will require vision, leadership, and some very hard decisions.

WE ARE ALL ONE

Despite the deepening political divisions within the country and across the globe, we need to begin to think beyond the local and regional end of things, especially when we are thinking of long-term strategies to better medicine and further its service to humanity. We need to look beyond the local landscape and target obstacles at the global level. We need to think beyond just communicable diseases and begin to tap into solving the scourge of noncommunicable diseases such as cancer and heart disease. There are going to be many barriers of unimaginable magnitude that we will have to strive to overcome. In the post-COVID aftermath, we have recognized that many of our larger institutions nose-dived and botched an opportune moment to show leadership. The response at the federal, state, and municipal levels was variable and, in many instances, unpredictable and untrustworthy. What enabled us to survive so far and will continue to serve us well has been our human spirit, resilience, and love for life. The world, however, will never be the same. The economic pain from the war on the virus and the war between us as humans is not going to go away quickly. It will take many years for global economies and the health care industry to recover.

As we realize that the crisis efforts at hospitals brought together cadres of individuals across health care organizations that had never before worked with each other, we get a sense that we are capable of a lot more collectively than we ever could have imagined. What will and what should health care look like for us over the next few years? Disease at one end of the globe can affect well-being and the economy at the other end. This interdependence and vulnerability extend beyond communicable diseases to lifestyle diseases like cancer and cardiovascular disease. And we all know for sure that much of the latter has been influenced by us in the West. We are all connected.

As much as we feel that walling ourselves off may be the solution, it could not be further from the truth. The survival of the world economic order and the health care industry is dependent on continuous connectivity and movement across the borders. As alluded to earlier, the barriers around reimbursement, regulatory hurdles, and providing care across state and international borders will go away. And that will happen because patients will drive it in that direction. So now is the time to recalibrate. What is essential versus nonessential, and high value versus low value, needs to be argued and resolved. Anything that is uneconomic in the new world order will be questioned and winnowed out.

Clearly, domestic and international health has become a number-one priority, especially after seeing how it can devastate the world economy acutely and with long-term effects. It has been succinctly stated by many during the pandemic that if you don't have healthy people, there is no health in the economy. It is humbling to be reminded that only 15 percent of health is affected by health care delivered. The rest of it lies within the social construct that directly determines and influences health. Creating pathways to overcome the inequities of the past and lay the framework to prevent those in the future is the need of the hour. Technology remains the only glimmer of hope. This is where digital strategies, aided by sensor advances, coupled with data sharing, and fueled by artificial intelligence will allow us to come together as one, to combat sicknesses even before they develop. For that we must ensure that the connectedness we are seeking is unbiased and all-encompassing.

18

HOSPITAL OF THE FUTURE

Technology has to become the connective tissue that holds together the continuum of care.
DAVID RUTHVEN

Sofia is a forty-two-year-old mother of three young children who is scheduled for elective abdominal surgery for colon cancer. About four weeks ago, she began experiencing severe abdominal pain and constipation that forced her to seek a consultation with her primary care physician. An iPhone colorimetric test followed by abdominal imaging showed that she had developed a large tumor encasing her colon, which was causing the pain and impeding her bowel movements. She was diagnosed with advanced colon cancer. She was shocked beyond belief, as there was no family history of cancer and she had been healthy all these years with no risk factors for any disease, let alone cancer. She was not even in the recommended age-group for regular colonoscopies and cancer screening.

She could now vaguely recollect that she had been feeling a sense of fullness in her belly for more than six months and had lost twelve pounds over this period, but had not made too much of that. In fact, she was quite pleased by the weight loss. Now here she was with this cancerous growth in her abdomen, which she was told had not yet spread but was too large to remove by minimally invasive surgery. Her symptoms continued to get much worse; she progressively got weaker and now felt nauseous all the time. Looking after herself and her young family had become a chore. She needed surgery soon. She needed an exploratory laparotomy with a wide resection of the colonic mass and the areas of healthy colon around it.

Let's look around the corner, at how care might look for her a few years from now. This speculative projection of the hospital care pathway could be the case for any form of elective, scheduled surgery, be it spinal surgery, a hernia repair, a cholecystectomy, heart surgery, brain surgery, or a radical prostatectomy.

Sofia is scheduled for surgery, and two weeks prior to her being admitted to the hospital, she receives a live video call from a health care navigator, Anita, welcoming her and identifying herself as the point person for any questions or concerns that may arise during Sofia's hospitalization. She explains to Sofia that she will begin to receive educational material in the form of video information capsules on her phone or computer, giving her preoperative instructions and contacts for any questions that she may have. She will also be connected with a digital community of prior patients with colon cancer who have been through the same procedure, who have volunteered their time to help answer personal queries that Sofia may have. This is the evolving "digital community of patients" who are experts at having lived with the disease and will be a part of the caregiving team, being there to interact in person as and when needed.

Three days prior to her scheduled admission, her personal check-engine light has been turned on for monitoring. She has routine monitoring initiated through a suite of mail-in sensors. She does not need a preoperative check, as the sensors have been tracking her heart rate, blood pressure, temperature, oxygen saturations, lung functions (via voice and spirometry), blood glucose, and other markers (natriuretic peptides) of her heart function. Besides this, her mobile ECG is being tracked, which gives insight into her blood electrolytes, predicts heart-rhythm abnormalities, and helps quantify her risk for death or any perioperative complications. The day before her procedure, she receives a live video call from an advanced care practitioner, who explains to her how the next few days in the hospital will look for her. Along with this, Sofia receives a "digital pass" with a welcome video outlining the layout of the hospital and her room, introducing her caregivers, providing a live map guiding her to her room, and showing the itemized schedule.

Sofia has a sense of calmness. No fear of the unknown, as she knows what to expect. When she arrives, the tranquility, the hospital layout, and the ergonomic design of her spacious hospital room further reinforce her confidence in the care that she is set to receive. Her furniture and bed have built-in sensors that seamlessly monitor and take her vital signs and other meaningful measurements. These are directly documented in her electronic medical record. She has a large video screen on her wall that will allow her to talk with her multiple doctors at the same time, and her kids and family. She can even access her records on the screen along with educational video materials. Everything is voice activated, including the virtual assistant device by her bedside, giving her instant access to the nursing station, the administration, the kitchen, or a health care professional. No trying to remember phone numbers or pressing call buttons and waiting for an eternity. The answers to any questions pertinent to the diagnosis, procedure, length of stay, and medication schedules are immediately available.

The digital wristband she was provided on arrival contains all her private information and can be scanned passively to confirm her identity before any investigation or procedure. The digital band is studded with sensors and can track her physical activity along with oxygen saturations and other vital signs that are connected to the network in her room, which in turn is automatically uploaded to her records. The data is continuous, as is the care. Variations from the baseline pattern above a set threshold are being processed by a built-in AI system ready to alert the nursing staff. Sofia can always access her own information.

She is surprised by a robot sliding from room to room delivering medications and supplies. A portable CT scan machine is wheeled into her room, and the resulting high-resolution image is used to construct a 3D-printed model of her abdominal organs and colon that will help the surgeon with the surgical procedure. This offers a reference model that can be used by her operating surgeon, providing alternative views of the colon that could serve to decrease the time and cost in the operating room and help improve recovery. At the same time, it is used as a teaching tool to give her a sense of what the procedure entails. All this is being done without her having to step outside her room.

Post-procedurally, after a short stint in the recovery unit, she is back in her room, which has been transformed into one capable of giving intensive-level care. All routine charting and orders are digitally uploaded via voice capture. When the attending doctor and team arrive, an overhead camera seamlessly captures the RFID tags on their identity badges, displaying their names and photographs on the large TV screen, making the introductions effortless. The doctor can pull up images from the surgery on the large screen without a keyboard click—it's all voice activated. The discussion is automatically processed by the built-in AI and transcribed into a note in the EMR. Discharge planning is done using her individualized data points across specific time points of her hospital stay with predictive analytics, helping to decide whether home, rehab, or a skilled-nursing facility is her next destination. Sofia is going home. Two days post–major surgery, she is going to recover at home, in her own bed. The home-hospital transition has been very smooth. She has a team of caregivers deputed to look after her as she recovers. The setup for home care is essentially the same: virtual care, sensors, risk stratification and warning systems, voice-activated virtual assistants, and a video screen remain the backbone of her care, all provided by the home-hospital team. During recovery she interacts with the health care team in person and virtually. Her physiotherapy and rehabilitation plan, initially in person, transitions quickly to a remote (digital) program.

Compare this to the disjointed, unpredictable, and clunky present-day experience: the multiple check-in lines; the missed phone calls; voice mails, answering machines, and telephone tag; disgruntled clinicians and secretaries; losing your way and seeking directions within the hospital maze; a prolonged inpatient stay; disrupted sleep, with frequent in-person collection of vital signs; missed meals; multiple hits and misses in meeting the consultants and specialists; getting the right information; impersonal, muddled discharge instructions; and mostly the fear of the unknown in a foreign environment.

THE NEED FOR CHANGE

The hospital is like a living, pulsatile, dynamic, multicellular organism. For it to survive, it depends on a coordinated and connected subcellular apparatus. The hospital of the future needs all the present-day siloed units connected within and outside the concrete structure. Sensors on, in, and around the patient transmitting data in real time, allowing for quality monitoring, individualized interventions, and resource-allocation optimization constitute the nodes and the connective tissue holding everything together. The hospital of the future will look very different from the way it is now. Those designing and building new structures must plan for a future that they may not yet fully understand. But it is the right time to rethink how hospitals need to look and operate in the immediate and intermediate future.

Health care continues to transform on a weekly basis as a result of cost concerns, quality issues, and legislative reform. Reactive changes account for instability and insecurity, and it is time for the entire health system to reinvent the business model at its core. Small, iterative steps will no longer cut it. Either you are all in or you're not. Some of this transformation has already commenced in the peri-pandemic period and lays the foundation for building the future. We even have a chance to take a shot at fixing the inequity of care across the planet. It is important that we take the helm here, rethink the hospital, and institute change. The adage still holds true: if you don't create change, change will create you.

RETHINKING THE HOSPITAL?

Today's hospitals are set up to fail. Their fiscal future is bleak. The operational inefficiencies and inability to embrace patients of all walks of life, in and outside the hospital, make the current system and its viability destined for a breakdown. When discussing the future, it is imperative to remember that it remains a moving target, and there can be many dystopian and impractical representations of how it may look. To be realistic and practical, this dialogue will target a time frame of five to ten years, keeping in mind that it may need to be open-ended—especially since circumstances will continually change, and the next best thing will always be just around the corner. Over the last couple of years, I have had innumerable conversations with hospital leaders and CEOs of several organizations. There are a variety of vantage points across those making the decisions, but there is consistency in the recognition of the impact of the advancing digital landscape and its influence on the delivery of care—the bottom line being that the hospital of the future will be reflective of who we are, what our priorities are, and what we want patient care to look like.

The hospital will evolve iteratively to be able to provide continuous care with a centralized digital center to assist in making collective team-based multispecialty decisions with or without the aid of AI-assisted algorithms. In the background, on-demand integration of virtual, sensor, and AI-driven technology aided by a system within an ambient intelligent environment will determine the shape of the workflow. The hospital framework will be like that of the central nervous system: a central command (like the higher cortical centers) with dendritic connections to multiple nodes across the hospital, enabling care from hospital entry to exit and beyond.

Gone are the days of a hospital building comprised of just concrete walls, partitioned into rooms for patients, procedures, and offices. As the architecture of any hospital evolves, it should do so with a clear idea of what it stands for, the promise it hopes to deliver, and providing the infrastructure for innovation seamlessly intertwined with the daily operations. The building sets the tone for a place of healing that is patient-centric. Everything within those four walls will reflect an environment of teamwork, multidisciplinary care with the focus being to enhance the patient experience while improving outcomes. Hospitals will have wellness-based designs with features promoting health. The space and lighting configuration will use nontoxic materials to engender a sense of well-being. The environment will inherently promote research, education, and a sense of community and connectedness.

Becoming a digital organization means weaving the culture into the organizational strategy, operations, and processes. Flexibility and scalability are central to the implementation process, especially if one has to endure and win the long game. Designs to promote physical, spiritual, and mental health while contributing to recovery will be essential. Spacious visitor lounges, healing gardens, ambient lighting with changing tones, a noise-free environment, and changing wall colors to promote well-being will become a part of the patient experience.

THE CARE CULTURE MAKEOVER

Culture is often dictated or incentivized by economics. For as long as I can remember, the focus of administrative leaders has been on turnover, reduced inpatient days, and length of stay. This is largely to keep the bean counters content, as patient turnover and throughput seem to be essential determinants of fiscal health. The pressure to make health care affordable and profitable is constant, as contradictory to each other as these two ideologies might seem. The answer lies in finding the right balance. Despite the concept of value-based care being floated around for the last decade, the gravitation in that direction has been gradual at best, with investments in digital care even slower. In what has always been a margin-compromised environment, investing in new technology has always meant appropriating resources away from conventional care. The hospital CEOs keep hoping that a federal government–sponsored fiscal incentive will get this underway, while the Centers for Medicare & Medicaid Services (CMS) and other federal bodies are happy to hold the status quo. Both forms of leadership are playing the waiting game and trying to stare each other down. Hence the inertia. There has been a feigned apathy from both sides, despite recognizing the call for action. And then COVID-19 struck, and an element of immediacy followed.

The hospital of the future will be shaped by the evolution of clinical care. Much of this transformation is occurring outside the four walls of the hospital, and we need to be ready to embrace it and bring it in. The hospital will reflect not a building or a facility but rather an ecosystem. The construct of the place will in turn influence the behavior and culture of the workforce. With the wide availability of smartphones, apps with the possibility of massive scalability through the cloud infrastructure will eliminate the clutter. The backbone will be lean thinking reinforced by predictive analytics. The road map to the structure of clinical care will in turn be determined by technological advancement and adoption. As discussed in much of this book, there will be an interplay of machine learning, virtual care, and mHealth powered by sensors at the front end. This will extend to easy and constant access for quick questions, urgent care, behavioral issues, outpatient care, and hospital-at-home initiatives enabling the transition of lower-acuity patients from the hospital to the home. It's not a question of why or how anymore, but of when.

COMMAND CENTERS

It won't be long before, analogous to the airline industry, every hospital system will have a central command station. This will begin by serving the purpose of being more efficient, using the in-hospital beds more resourcefully and effectively; managing administrative tasks such as delivery of medicines, linen, or food in a centralized way; overseeing the use of space in the outpatient arena; and adjusting the flow between procedural and operating rooms. Beyond this, the central command station will help provide individualized care, charting the flight paths of patients and disease management platforms, examining trends and deviations, and enabling proactive care. These clinical command centers will provide uninterrupted information (through sensors) on the clinical state, risk factors, and trajectory. Machine-learning approaches will help cluster patient groups, facilitating redistribution of care and allocation of resources to specific patient areas in real time. The use of predictive analytics will further abet administrative tasks such as interfacility transfers while better managing length of stay and discharges.

An essential part of the infrastructure is to ensure that the ecosystem should not be all about finances and throughput. It should facilitate discovery while cultivating the environment for data-driven basic and clinical science that will lead to novel treatment strategies. The research infrastructure needs to be broadened to enable a multidisciplinary translational and collaborative approach. The hospital command center being fed all this digital data will allow risk stratification of patient populations early in the disease states, often in the subclinical state to manage, track, enroll in clinical trials, and improve outcomes. It behooves us to create a hospital infrastructure that is linked to the disease management platforms that track patients through their life cycle into the outpatient world. This will not only enhance care continuity but allow us to become smarter at leveraging technology to monitor outcomes, adherence, adverse effects of medicines, or late complications from a surgical procedure.

One big, recurrent theme is alarm fatigue. You walk into a telemonitoring unit and you can hear alarms constantly going off, with little response from the staff. It's simply a case of desensitization. Providers can experience up to two hundred alarms per bed per day, with 99 percent of these literal false alarms. AI allows an automated way of categorizing these alarms, reducing false notifications, and thereby reducing staff fatigue. A central-command strategy will help by enabling a more judicious use of resources and personnel for monitoring patients.

THE FLEXIBLE FUTURE STATE

Traditional care is inefficient and expensive. Care outside the hospital, or lack thereof, often determines the need for in-hospital care. The interdependence of these two major components of the life cycle of every individual will serve to inspire how clinical medicine and the hospital of the future need to evolve. Flexibility will result from the use of technology within and outside the hospital that will work to ease the pressure points on the continuity of care while enhancing efficiency and cutting costs.

The hospital structure will have the ability to constantly evolve in tandem with medicine that is morphing on a day-to-day basis. The framework of such a construct will be built with digital bricks. Technology will hold together care as it is delivered now and how it will be in the future. The scaffold we create will serve to replicate the nervous system of the human body. Command centers reflective of the human brain will be seamlessly connected to patients and sensors in and outside the hospital. Embedded data-monitoring centers will continually provide feedback to patients, encouraging self-learning. AI-assisted algorithms embolden self-management. The key components of the future hospital state will include a few essentials. The first, which has been talked about a lot already, is precision medicine, where care will be individualized using sensors and artificial intelligence. The second is focused on enhancing the patient experience, which will be a seamless digital one, punctuated with human contact at precise nodes to prevent care from becoming an impersonal interaction. There will be incremental iterative steps toward automation. To start with, this automation will be dedicated to enhancing operational efficiencies via use of robotics, supply chains, blockchain, and AI-assisted backend enhancements. As the low-hanging fruits of repetitive administrative tasks get expunged, active patient management complementing conventional in-person care to enhance the patient experience and outcomes will become the primary focus.

With the unremitting use of handhelds and smartphones and continuous streaming data, it will be impossible to get the best out of telemedicine and sensor approaches without fully embracing a digital framework. Also, increasing patient expectations and empowerment make it imperative that the hospital of the future be built on a platform that enables flexibility and allows the system to be nimble. As stated earlier, it will be this digital framework that extends beyond the hospital structure to help erase the existing digital divide for those who are currently disenfranchised and marginalized by socioeconomic factors.

Having a digital framework in place will be central to the implementation of technological innovations as they continue to evolve at a breathtaking pace. Abnormal laboratory values (integrated with data from the EMR) will trigger an AI application to automatically send out an invitation for a virtual or in-person clinic appointment. Chatbot-facilitated communication between patients and clinical staff will become the norm, as digital platforms connect patients and providers. Anyone with a smartphone will be able to connect with their smart hospital through a collection of mobile apps. This digital platform will have the flexibility to be upgraded with the ever-increasing array of sensors, the goal being to keep patients healthier, engaging them in their own care aided by precision medicine, and diminishing the need for hospital-based inpatient care. Or, for that matter, even hospital-based outpatient care. The evolution of the hospital of the future will be configured by the changing demographics, aging population, and economic imperative to obtain better value for health care.

THE BED PARADOX

They say it's all about the beds. Balancing the right number of beds with the right extent of resources can keep hospitals profitable and solvent; however, what is that right number? Notably, there are and always will be regional, national, and international differences between hospitals as to what that number should actually be. Prior to the pandemic, MedPAC (an independent body reporting to Congress) stated that there are more hospital beds in the United States than actually needed. In support of this statement, in years preceding the pandemic, a flurry of hospitals closed. This does seem significantly incongruous with lived experiences within many academic tertiary centers, where there is forever a bed crunch.

Teams of doctors, nurses, and administrators struggle on a daily basis to move patients around to free up beds to accept emergent transfers. A large part of this is due to the lack of real-time information and the absence of sophisticated systems engineering and analytics to use the beds more efficiently. The pandemic has certainly already shifted outpatient care to the home, and we can also envisage a part of inpatient care becoming home-centered. The inpatient environment is likely to change in the coming years, where the hospital will largely constitute a boarding and treatment center for the sickest of the sick, as discharges will decrease and length of stays will increase. The hospital will more likely than not become a clunky, expensive cost center, and its viability will depend on the ability to be engaged in services and innovations across the complete life cycle of the patient between home to the hospital and back.

AI and machine learning will enable forecasting health care demands across hospitals and regions. This will be across the spectrum of emergency or inpatient needs, virtual or in-person encounters, further empowering health systems to refine markets and set strategy. Importantly, analytics will be a dynamic exercise rather than an intermittent and periodic undertaking. There will be a unique flexibility within the system to adapt to where, when, and what the need may be. Flexible design constructs between the outpatient and inpatient areas will allow for stepping up the bed count if needed in an emergency.

WHAT WILL INPATIENT CARE LOOK LIKE?

The brick-and-mortar facade may appear the same, but internally the operations will be quite different. The inpatient experience will involve telemedicine, ambient sensor technology, and artificial intelligence inclusive of natural language processing to make the entire stay friction-free. The video platform already made it into the patient room during the pandemic; iPads allowed the health care providers to interact with the patient without stepping into their room. This, combined with the objective parameters of health gleaned from sensors within the room, will make the interaction meaningful and quantitative. Ambient technology with the use of virtual assistants will enable the physician to have a detailed discussion with the patient, with the automatic creation of a visit note that populates in the EMR.

Inpatient rooms will be personalized to accommodate families, technology, and voice-activated video screens. No wires, no tethering to the bed, the monitor, or to intravenous stands. Vital signs and other relevant data will be wirelessly collected from sensors embedded in the walls, furniture, television screen, and the bed. The rooms will have vents with sensors to monitor the air, and detect and report an airborne infection. Large video screens will allow for conversations with multiple clinicians and family members at the same time, along with a live display of clinical data and test results. This way the medical oncologist, surgeon, radiologist, social worker, pharmacy, and radiation oncologist can all simultaneously meet with the patient and the family and have a constructive discussion to reach a consensus on next steps.

As much of ambulatory care shifts to patients' homes, some of the existing inpatient care will shift to the ambulatory arena or will become home-based with more refined monitoring. This will be necessary as Big Data directs the transformation of a fee-for-service system into a value-based one. Inpatient care will become a collective value-based team sport of multiple clinicians working together to provide the most efficient individualized care. Continuous data will mandate continuous care, and the digital framework will enable that, while also improving the patient experience and efficiency within the hospital. Machine learning to detect bottlenecks and under- and overuse of operating times and rooms will also be tracked. Using mobile technology, surgeons and interventionalists will release, request, or swap time blocks as needed. Medical equipment will continue to get smaller and more portable. This will enable most imaging (inclusive of CT) and procedures at the bedside. Care will be brought to the patient, rather than the other way around. Care will be mobile.

Future hospital systems will leverage the internet of things (IoT) to the hilt. Along with integrating information from multiple sources, this could also serve as an early notification system. Machine intelligence platforms will collect data from sensors embedded in the beds, furniture, ceilings, building systems, and clinical apps, along with those from the patient monitors serving to risk-stratify, and notify the clinical team of any problematic findings. Beyond individualized care, this also provides a surveillance system that permits better operational support. Early warning systems to alert hospital administrators and caregivers will facilitate more resource-appropriate care and outcomes. An IoT- and AI-facilitated connectivity will disrupt the conventional modus operandi. This new age is around the corner.

HOME-BASED CARE

When seventy-eight-year-old Jim Lee was told that he had an infected heart valve and would require six weeks of antibiotics, he took the news in stride. When I told him that he would have to receive this as an inpatient, he nearly broke down. He could not fathom being cooped up in the hospital or a skilled-nursing facility for six weeks. He lived alone with his yellow Labrador, Skip, and had no way of ensuring that Skip could be looked after while he recovered from his infection. This is just one simple story among countless others that happen every day, of people confronted with the decision of having to be admitted to a hospital and figuring out a way to fend for themselves and loved ones during that period of confinement. Home-based care is already happening for a variety of conditions, such as the administration of antibiotics, wound management, home hospice, and so on. This was not new. But Jim had a slew of other comorbidities and illnesses that made present-day home-based care challenging. His kidneys were at the brink of failing, and he had developed heart failure that needed close, steady monitoring. If we had the right suite of sensors, coupled with remote monitoring and patient-centric care, it could be different. We know that one-third of the elderly above the age of seventy and more than half of those older than eighty leave the hospital more disabled than when they entered it. Add to this a cohort of patients at the end stages of their lives who spend most of their time traveling to and from the hospital, sometimes several hours a day, when they could be at home focusing on things that are more important to them.

It goes without saying that most of us would rather be at home than in the hospital. Most patients dislike hospitals, for a variety of reasons; the smell, the food, the aura, the anxiety that it provokes are just a few. We also know that medical errors in the hospital setting are the third largest cause of death after cancer and heart disease, besides the risk of getting a hospital-acquired infection. If we could provide hospital-level care at home, that would be the holy grail. This care at home needs to mirror the care provided in the hospital in terms of daily clinical evaluation, assessment of vital signs and laboratory tests, intravenous medications, food services, and speech and physical therapy. Hospitals are also already setting up programs where digital technology will enable patients to be monitored in their own homes. If sensors can report objectively on patients in real time and blood and urine tests can be performed using smartphones and connecting devices, this would enable more cost-effective care in a preferred location. Some of the most common conditions, such as congestive heart failure, chronic obstructive lung disease, urinary tract infections, pneumonia, and cellulitis can now be managed more cost-effectively in your preferred environment.

For example, the cost of pneumonia treatment within a hospital environment can be ten to twenty times more than at home, and still we see many cases of mild pneumonia getting admitted to the hospital. Many of these patients are low risk and could easily be treated at home, not to mention that hospitalization itself carries risks of iatrogenic complications and other hospital-acquired infections, many of which could be avoided. Home health care solutions have evolved to a level that their implementation has already begun—but in a limited way. As science fiction writer William Gibson prophetically stated, “The future is already here, it’s just not evenly distributed.”

For some places, these practices have begun. Patients with dehydration, pneumonias, cellulitis, or other low-risk conditions are often now sent home with intravenous lines in place, with visiting nurse and hospital-at-home services. Several hospitals now have such programs in place, which provide monthlong care and set up patients with services to avoid readmissions. There is a move to expand these programs to conventional in-hospital routine post-operative care. It is highly likely that the in-hospital recovery will continue to be further abbreviated, and that a sizable component of the early recovery period will be at home. Patients who have just had cardiac surgery and are out of the ICU may not have to spend a week in the intermediate care environment in the hospital, but instead will be shifted home with the right kinds of services. Even chemotherapy will be administered at home, ensuring a sense of normalcy while allaying the anxiety, depression, and stress that accompanies the hospital environment. It has been estimated that one-third of overall care provided in the hospital will be shifted home in the coming years. When it comes to chronic diseases, almost half the care for these conditions will be managed at home. Obviously, the pathways of remote care will need to be carefully curated and tested in a variety of clinical use cases.

Hospitals are going asset-light, with patient homes becoming a part of the hospital inpatient or outpatient estate. It is becoming possible for a patient to receive hospital-like care in their very own home. Biosensors in the bedroom, with a constant transmission of vital signs coupled with other relevant physiologic metrics, can replace the in-hospital, cursory check. Objective quantifiable data from the sensors, along with apps that can aid a detailed physical exam, will further add value. Smart medical homes to look after the elderly and the frail through sensor-based approaches to monitoring mobility, activities of daily living, and falls will further shorten hospital stays and reduce the time in nursing homes before moving patients to their own home, while smart pillboxes and RFID strategies will help monitor adherence. This will be further accompanied by a cadre of remote health care providers, leading to fewer boots on the ground in the hospital campus. The issues of privacy and autonomy will come up, as well as whether the home-care extension is scalable across all communities and socioeconomic strata. There are already efforts to construct an Airbnb-like model for out-of-hospital home care. Churches, temples, and community centers could become a part of this schema to provide out-of-hospital care to the homeless and disenfranchised.

The hospital of the future will be incentivized to have fewer beds and instead set up state-of-the-art remote-monitoring centers, enabling these home-hospital programs to become an extension of the hospital framework. There will be modular components, where conventional inpatient or specialized care can be administered through systems at home or rural ambulatory-care sites. This would be akin to well-oiled disease management platforms that cover the inpatient-outpatient life span. It is worth mentioning that as much as in-hospital beds will shrink within community hospitals, it probably won't be the same case in tertiary and quaternary care centers. There will need to be a place to look after the really sick patients, where they will most likely stay admitted for longer periods than previously.

A few years ago, in an interview with the *Wall Street Journal*, Dr. Kenneth Davis, Mount Sinai's president and chief executive, was asked about concerns about reducing the number of hospital beds, especially should there be a citywide emergency. Dr. Davis said, "We can't build facilities for doomsday. We need a model of care that focuses on wellness and prevention and keeps people out of hospitals." A great model to aspire for (as we should)—but look what happened. We had an unparalleled pandemic that exposed the kinks in the current system and our vision for the future. After we recover from this, it will happen again. Whether the next crisis is a pandemic, natural disaster, or war, an essential prerequisite is a system that is nimble and flexible enough to adapt to the needs and scalable enough to accommodate the demands of humanity. Allowing for hospital space that can be flexed into crisis or pandemic mode is essential. This would mean parking garages, foyers, and reception areas could be easily converted into triage and holding areas, while office spaces, in-hospital corridors, and lobby areas could accommodate extra beds and increased inpatient volume. We need to begin planning accordingly.

STAFFING

Staffing within this ecosystem will continue to evolve. Advanced clinical practitioners, including physician assistants and nurse practitioners, will play a leadership role within the framework of these remote-monitoring setups as we wait for the deep-learning algorithms to aid and abet this new world order. Job descriptions for physicians will also change. Besides the conventional practice, physicians across all specialties will be available 24-7 to provide remote consultative services as needed. This will be coupled with an increase in home nursing and specialist support, all driven by patient expectations.

Predictive analytics will help review data, improve efficiency, and recommend algorithm-driven interventions along with the use of intelligent staffing. This will allow physician assistants and nurse practitioners to delegate responsibility to RNs and health care navigators, helping everyone to work at the top of their license. This is the era of health care navigators, who will serve to provide the personalized care that is currently missing. They will help with triaging, providing education, answering queries, and managing patients using directed algorithms.

With the incorporation of remote care, the scheduling for clinicians will be personalized to prevent burnout and shortages. Retirements will decrease, as older physicians interested in continuing to practice could do so by being available to be a part of this new workforce focusing on the remote delivery of care. AI will help us analyze the supply-and-demand patterns and ensure better utilization of the workforce to provide access to patients as and when they need it. It is quite likely that these remote-monitoring centers may not be in close proximity to the concrete building but will still lie within the umbrella of the digital scaffold. Depending on institutional aspirations and scalability of the efforts, the footprint and geography of hospitals will extend beyond state and national borders. It is through this that the digitally enabled hospital of the future will help address the issue of health equity. This does not take away the fact that hospitals will still need to have the infrastructure to provide cutting-edge cancer therapies, sophisticated neurosurgery, complex cardiovascular surgical interventions, and novel therapies across the different disciplines while providing acute and intensive care.

AMBULATORY CARE

The quick adoption of telehealth during the early months of the pandemic was quite telling. It showed that a significant proportion of patients could be evaluated remotely through telemedicine. Even though at the end of every surge there was an uptick of in-person visits, the pendulum will swing toward a hybrid strategy. A substantial proportion of conventional outpatient care will move to telecare. The digital framework of the hospital structure will expand into the homes of our patients. Outpatient offices from within the core structure of the hospital will shift to ambulatory sites away from the main hospitals and closer to the community. These offices will consist of medically smart rooms with infrastructure and IT systems to assist the clinicians with monitoring and treatment in person and remotely as requested. The impact of sensors and artificial intelligence in this setting has been discussed in detail in earlier sections. Even though in-person and telehealth visits may be periodically scheduled, the surveillance through sensors during this in-between phase will be continuous. Virtual care will help transform outpatient appointments into one-stop visits with multidisciplinary teams of clinicians all Zooming in for the visit.

As in Sofia's case, sensors will transpose the outpatient laboratory to the patient living room. Automatic downloads of vital signs, weight, and blood pressure will complement a virtual clinic visit to focus on the problem at hand. The wait time before and after the visit will be eliminated, as will travel, traffic, parking, elevators, and the waiting room. Self-management will be a big part of the construct of the futuristic hospital. There will need to be creative solutions and resources to empower patients to take on their own care. Patients will have a shared responsibility toward achieving their outcomes, using patient-specific dashboards with a clear delineation of their daily, monthly, and yearly goals displayed on their health care portal. These could be lifestyle, vital signs, dietary, or disease-specific goals such as an achievable blood pressure, cholesterol, or hemoglobin A1C level. A combination of high technology with high touch will translate into high-quality care with better patient outcomes. Individuals not following a predicted clinical course will have enough medical, sociodemographic, and genetic data to enable the determination of the reason for the variance. Future care in the ambulatory setting will be exemplified by ambient, intelligent computing that can respond in real time. Sensors will passively collect information in the background. These sensors could be at home, the office, the car, or on the person. The data from various sensors will work through the IoT in an all-in-one fashion, generating individual specific data and algorithms.

It is important to emphasize that human contact and in-person clinic visits should and will always remain an integral part of the system of care. There is much that can be missed in tele-visits, especially in the absence of objective data from sophisticated sensor strategies. The evolution of ambulatory care will evolve in a graded manner, mostly driven by digital innovations. These ambulatory outpatient sites will be small, friendly, and more comfortable, not intimidating like the enormity of the quaternary structure within which they are embedded as of today. Secondary care, inclusive of procedures, will largely be shifted away from the main campuses. The payment system will evolve to enable this to happen. Hospitals will be incented by the acuity of care that allows them to match the right patient to the right place. End-of-life care will be either at centers set up for this or at home. This would not be merely to balance the fiscal equation and reduce costs, but to do the right thing toward preserving human dignity and improving the patient experience.

The in-person outpatient experience will be seamless. Scheduling will be online. There will be no registration, just a digital pass. Phone, facial, or digital print recognition will become the norm. Much of this is AI-enabled and already finding its way into stadiums and airports. Blood tests will be done through an adapter on the phone at home or in person with robotic assistance in the phlebotomy lab.

PATIENT EXPERIENCE

One can imagine the patient experience of the future proceeding from an interaction with a chatbot or a symptom checker that facilitates the triage of the patient to an appropriate clinician, who is available on-demand for consultation. This visit will first be a virtual encounter that will help the doctor address the issue at hand. If there is something that needs immediate clinical attention, then even prior to the virtual visit there could be an instantaneous call to an ambulance or even a rideshare app that would bring the patient to the clinic or to the hospital.

This will be an integrated, seamless experience, in which all the conventional hurdles related to appointments and insurance coverage will be automatically handled via AI algorithms at the backend. This digital encounter would not be one of repeated phone calls, call waiting, robot assistance that puts patients on a never-ending loop. This digital-door access could provide patient care through the entire life cycle of the disease. It could follow the patient from an outpatient environment to the urgent-care clinic and a hospital admission, from inpatient care to rehab and subsequently to their next outpatient visit.

The health sector is beginning to align with other industries, namely, retail and finance, which are most responsive to the needs of the consumer, with a greater number of choices. The imminence of having medical care fit into our everyday life and not the other way around is going to become important. Patient satisfaction and outcomes will become key drivers for reimbursement. Virtual assistants are already finding their way into hospital rooms, with an ability to answer most frequently asked questions, such as those related to discharge time, visitor rules, payment plans, coverage, and rehabilitation instructions.

Although patients over sixty-five represent 16 percent of the population, they comprise nearly half of hospitalized patients. The elderly population continues to grow, and by 2030, one in every five Americans will be over the age of sixty-five. Patients admitted to the hospital will continue to be older and with more complex needs, with the care continuum and patient experience needing to extend beyond the four walls of the hospital into their homes. This will encompass the preadmission period all the way through long-term care. The goal will be to create an environment where the patient's family and caregivers are encouraged to work together and communicate inside and outside the hospital's walls. The hospital of the future will have invested in partnerships with ride, food delivery, and community services. As care begins to extend beyond state borders and national boundaries, patients will seek out caregivers and hospitals based on value, performance, and reputation.

There will be institutional moves to use consumer analytics to create targeted engagement strategies for patients across different disease states and demographic distributions. As we step onto this path of AI and automation with trepidation, we will embark on a journey of discovery and exploration. Sensors and AI will become as ubiquitous as wireless networks. But this is not going to be easy; it will take a lot of hard work. In what is today a resource-constrained environment, it may seem counterintuitive to invest in technology, but there is no way out. It will pay back in dividends.

THE METAVERSE, ROBOTS, AND TAMING THE FUTURE

The metaverse is an integrated computer-generated network through which remote care will be provided as an immersive experience in a shared three-dimensional virtual environment. As described earlier, this will enable the treatment of mental health disorders and provide personalized postsurgical rehabilitation while assisting interventional and surgical procedures. As an example, radiological images from the CT or MRI can overlay the surgical field, providing details regarding where the scalpel should cut, the catheter be placed, or the prosthetic fitted. Beyond this, the metaverse will also enable multiple physicians to work together to treat a challenging clinical situation, surgeons to practice, and trainees to learn through gamification.

The metaverse furthers the promise of "digital twins." This twinning of the real person creates the ability to predict and prevent disease and enables experimenting with new therapies on the digital replica. Digital twins will enable fast-forwarding time to examine the impact of an intervention, or play back an unfortunate occurrence, or insert an intervention to see if it can change the clinical outcome. The metaverse will expand the reach of the hospital of the future while it edges toward the construct of a virtual hospital.

A few years ago, the conversation about robots in medicine may have appeared dystopian, but it has become a reality. Robots have always been a part of the grand vision of futuristic hospitals and can be simplistically categorized as surgical or nonsurgical. Besides helping manage patients and services, they can play a significant role in preventing, diagnosing, and treating disease. Robots with a sophisticated array of sensors and AI can be humanized and friendly.

Surgical robots have been in a state of development for many years. For a wide variety of surgical procedures involving the heart, abdomen, and thorax, and for cancer located all over the body, robot-assisted surgical interventions are coming to the forefront. The da Vinci surgical robot gives the surgeon precise control and makes exact and accurate incisions. Robotics have been used to assist laparoscopic techniques that are minimally invasive and use concomitant imaging to guide the robotic arms to the right spot with the highest level of precision. AI and sensors are built into the robotic limbs to enhance functionality. A system of lasers, sensors, and waypoints from internally stored maps via imaging allow the robots to navigate obstacles.

The cyber knife is a noninvasive robotic form of therapy that allows for the precise delivery of radiation therapy to submillimeter precision. This is especially useful for tumors in surgically complex regions such as the head, neck, prostate, and other lower abdominal organs. The Veebot is another robot designed to assist in drawing blood. An imaging-assisted approach helps the robot find the vein quickly and with high accuracy. This is a human-assisted approach, so a manual override is possible at any time. There are nanorobots that swim through our bloodstream and lymphatics. They are less than a few millimeters in size and can be used to deliver drugs or therapies in a targeted fashion. Origami robots are capsules that are swallowed and dissolve when they enter the stomach, releasing a robot. This can then be controlled with an external magnetic field and used to patch wounds within the stomach lining, deliver medicines, or remove objects.

Other robots can lift and move patients in and out of beds and wheelchairs and help patients stand from a recumbent position. These will progressively find a larger role in geriatric units and in quaternary hospitals that look after the sickest patients. Pharma-assist robots help with medication management and dispensing. These robots reduce the repetitive administrative tasks of storage and dispensing. This in turn enables the pharmacist to participate in the clinical care of the patient. The XDBOT is an extreme disinfectant robot developed in Singapore that can be controlled remotely. It is motorized with wheels and has a dexterous robotic arm that can mimic human movement. This allows for the arm to reach tough locations, nooks, and crannies to clean and spray disinfectants. It has a six-axis arm that can navigate using sensors and high-definition cameras controlled by a laptop or a tablet. There is also the PARO therapeutic robot, used to improve the quality of life during recovery from surgery or illnesses, as well as depression or mental health problems. This robot looks like a baby seal and provides animal therapy. It can respond by name, enjoys being stroked, can wiggle and blink, and makes funny noises. These robots make the patients happy and reduce stress and anxiety. In a makeshift hospital in Wuhan, China, during the pandemic, robots were deployed to disinfect hospital rooms, deliver meals, and even entertain patients. One humanoid medical robot, known as Cloud Ginger, was able to provide information to patients and entertain them with dancing. In the setting of the pandemic, robots were essential to minimize instances of contact between infected patients and medical staff, reducing exposure and risk for infection.

On the inpatient floors, it is well known that only a fraction of nursing time is spent in direct patient contact. Much of the time is in administrative tasks, ordering supplies and a host of other nonclinical work. Put all this together, and the need for robots to help with repetitive, mundane tasks that don't require a whole lot of human intellect is self-evident. On the service front, let's begin by acknowledging that the hospital is a complicated operation. There is a constant flow of people, patients, materials, food, drugs, supplies, linen, and goods from one end to the other. Depending on the size of the hospital, this can mean several hundred miles of travel over the course of a day or week. There is constant movement of supplies and goods between hospital rooms, storage areas, pharmacies, pantries, offices, operating theaters, laundries, and so on. The next-generation hospital will have robots for these various tasks, be they delivering food, collecting results, or transporting blood samples and medications. This will free up nurses' time and allow them to spend greater amounts of time engaged in clinical tasks. Hospitals will have to create an ecosystem that will enable autonomous robot operations. This will require some planning and forward thinking and may necessarily involve the construction of underground tunnels and dedicated pathways to facilitate automated delivery and the movement of robots through the hospital. Some hospitals already have a lineup of robots awaiting tasks. As one heads out, the next one slides into the vacated spot, ready for its turn. The robots can work their way to the appropriate loading bay, up and down elevators, and on to the appropriate location to deliver their supplies.

Nearly 50 percent of health care workers in the United States alone are planning to leave their positions by 2025, with a postulated global shortage of 12.9 million (an underestimation) by 2035. Robots will fill this shortage. The role of robots will continue to increase, replacing a select set of personnel engaged in repetitive and tedious tasks where possible. They are already delivering drugs and meals and carrying away medical waste and disinfecting floors and hospital rooms. There are also robots participating in clinic rounds, being used for remote visits, and assisting with consultations and training. Robots will become an essential part of the hospital staff but will always be supervised by humans.

Alan Kay, a legendary computer scientist, once said that the best way to predict the future is to invent it. The future of the hospital is tied to technological advancements and the integration of telemedicine, sensors, and artificial intelligence. Beyond just recognizing the inevitability of this future, we need to seize it and become enthusiastic partners. While caring for each other, it will be our collective responsibility to ensure that technology remains forever tamed and we preserve the human touch. As has been wisely stated, "Technology is a useful servant, but a dangerous master."

EPILOGUE

It's been more than three years since the onset of the pandemic in the US, with more than one million dead and a hundred million infected. I was one of the hundred million, but one of the fortunate ones—lucky enough to survive the virus and the long haul of sequelae and persistent symptoms, unlike several million others across the US and the globe. I have had to relive the COVID experience many times with friends and family, who have each had to face their own battles with this vicious bug. Over the past couple of years, I have tried to do my bit by serving on the front line, looking after patients with and without COVID.

This pandemic has taught us many lessons, but I already see the pendulum swinging back to where it started. Not all the way back, but far enough that we must remind ourselves not to make the same mistakes again. One could ascribe some of this to our natural inertia, our propensity to gravitate toward our comfort zone, but most of it can be blamed on an inflexible system that has too many stakeholders vested in the status quo. The system will continue to evolve, in part because of the innovative mindset of clinicians and researchers, but mostly because of the expectations of our patients.

We need to remain hopeful for the future, excited about new technology, but refrain from allowing ourselves to get hypnotized by the shiny gizmos and widgets. The slowing of the pace of advancement, although not intentional, may serve to be useful in making sure that we don't allow ourselves to be totally enamored of and consumed by technology. There are some fundamentals in the practice of medicine that need to be preserved not just for now, but for a lifetime. The greatest of these is the human element.

It is imperative that we use the uptick in digital health technology to our advantage but at the same time prevent care from becoming an algorithm-driven, impersonal experience. The human touch, empathy, and compassion can never be replaced, even by the highest level of artificial intelligence. The practice of medicine revolves around our humanness, it mirrors our deepest realities, and it should never be transformed into an exclusively digital experience. Outsourcing touch and conversation to the robot may not be a smart way to practice medicine. Sensor-aided virtual care powered by predictive analytics is here, but should be used as a complementary stratagem to the human connection between the clinician and the patient, not a replacement of that bond.

Clinical practice patterns may not change with the same furious pace as they did during the early months of the pandemic, but change they will. The technology will continue to advance, with the centerpiece being the patient, who will become the point of care. Diagnoses and treatments will come to the patient, wherever the patient may be . . . and that is the future.

ACKNOWLEDGMENTS

For someone who has written nothing but scientific papers for the last three decades, writing this book meant taking a journey through uncharted territory. It has truly been an amazing and fulfilling voyage with several ups and downs, and one that I could not have taken alone.

I started writing this book approximately a year before the onset of the pandemic. And then COVID came and disrupted all our lives. After my personal encounter with the virus, the book took on a new meaning to me. The catalytic effect that the pandemic had on digital health made what I thought was going to be futuristic into something contemporary. The importance of transforming our health care system into a personalized, sustainable one that can care for humans all over the world seemed like a worthy goal to pursue. Therein lies the premise of this book.

First, I am very grateful to my patients, who have always inspired me to think of a better way of doing things. All the stories I have told are true, but I have changed some details to preserve confidentiality.

I'd like to thank my parents, who have been instrumental in most key decisions in my life. My mother's continuous (often unsolicited) advice on the virtue of humility has set the tone for much of my life and consequently the stories in this book. My dad's restless energy and pursuit of new opportunities at every stage of his life, and his advice that we are not born to profess just one discipline in life, have inspired me time and again to sidestep the conventional academic mold. They have touched this book and my writings in more ways than one can imagine.

This book would never have seen the light of day without the love and encouragement of my children. My son, Ashan, and daughter, Ahaana, were there at every stage of this production—right from the early discussions through my tryst with COVID and each of the multiple rejections that I encountered at every turn. Even though they may have suspected on many occasions that their old man was on a crazy trip, they never once failed to cheer me on and direct me toward finding my true voice. They encouraged me to begin writing blogs to transform my writing style into one that was more readable. This was possible through Ahaana's continuous guidance, love, and hand-holding. She helped me find the right tone in my writing with her extensive red-lining of my early blogs. So if you don't like my style of writing, blame her.

I am very grateful to my friends, Harish Lecamwasam and Daniel Friedman, who took the time to read very early versions of this book and did not feel compelled to stop me. I must thank my sister-in-law, Rupa Raje Gupta, who read the first-ever draft of this book in its primordial form. She made it clear to me that I needed to overhaul my writing and my message if it was meant to reach a wider audience. Advice that I took to heart.

I can't forget Stuart Horwitz, who assisted and guided me in crafting the very first version of the book proposal. I am extremely grateful to my wonderful agent, Stacey Glick. Stacey saw potential in the proposal and in me, which gave me the confidence to continue to hold pen to paper and keep writing. She helped me further fine-tune and hone an exciting, futuristic, yet practical book proposal.

I am very lucky to have the best senior editor ever. I am ever so grateful to Daniela Rapp, who has been with me through every moment of putting this book together. She helped me focus on continuing to think big, while not forgetting to pay attention to the small things. She prodded me to step away from medical jargon and encouraged me to add new stories that would help the narrative for my readers. This book would not have been possible without her shepherding the project.

Finally, I must thank my wife, Noopur, the love of my life, who has had to endure the entirety of this tumultuous journey and my mood swings. I sometimes wonder whether she was just happy that I was keeping myself busy and out of her hair. Well, I must admit that without her, I would be nothing. I continue to push myself, hoping that one day I will impress her. Even this book will most likely fall short.

NOTES

INTRODUCTION

7 ***Simple measures of physical*** - Singh, J. P., et al. 2009. "Device Diagnostics and Long-Term Clinical Outcome in Patients Receiving Cardiac Resynchronization Therapy." *Europace* 11:1647–53.

7 ***More recently, I*** - Boehmer, J. P., et al. 2017. "A Multisensor Algorithm Predicts Heart Failure Events in Patients with Implanted Devices: Results from the MultiSENSE Study." *JACC Heart Fail* 5:216–25.

7 ***Such as heart failure exacerbations*** - Merchant, F. M., G. W. Dec, and J. P. Singh. 2010. "Implantable Sensors for Heart Failure." *Circ Arrhythm Electrophysiol* 3:657–67.

7 ***The identification*** - Gardner, R. S., et al. 2018. "HeartLogic Multisensor Algorithm Identifies Patients During Periods of Significantly Increased Risk of Heart Failure Events: Results from the MultiSENSE Study." *Circ Heart Fail* 11. e004669.

7 ***I have also used*** - Maille, B., et al. 2021. "Smartwatch Electrocardiogram and Artificial Intelligence for Assessing Cardiac-Rhythm Safety of Drug Therapy in the COVID-19 Pandemic. The QT-Logs Study." *Int J Cardiol* 331:333–39.

7 ***Creating a digital twin*** - Laubenbacher, R., et al. 2022. "Building Digital Twins of the Human Immune System: Toward a Roadmap." *npj Digit. Med.* 5:1–5.

7 ***This is where*** - Zhao, M., J. H. Wasfy, and J. P. Singh. 2020. "Sensor-Aided Continuous Care and Self Management: Implications for the Post-COVID Era." *Lancet Digit Health* 2:e632–e634.

8 ***The downstream impact*** - Chatterjee, N. A., and J. P. Singh. 2017. "Making Sense of Remote Monitoring Studies in Heart Failure." *Eur Heart J* 38:2361–63.

8 ***Deep structural changes*** - Singh, J. P. 2018. "Connecting Life with Devices." *JACC Clin Electrophysiol* 4:422–23.

OUR BIG, FAT, SICK HEALTH CARE SYSTEM: THE NEED FOR CHANGE

12 ***In hospitals across the US*** - Haymarket Media. 2016. "Wide Price Variability for Standard

Radiographic Imaging." *Rheumatology Advisor.* https://www.rheumatologyadvisor.com/home/general-rheumatology/wide-price-variability-for-standard-radiographic-imaging/.

12 ***While a head computed tomography (CT)*** - Bassett, M. 2014. "Analysis: High Costs, Price Variability Mean Imaging Should Be a Healthcare Savings Target." *Fierce Healthcare.* www.fiercehealthcare.com/it/analysis-high-costs-price-variability-mean-imaging-should-be-a-healthcare-savings-target.

12 ***It is inevitable*** - Wooldridge, S. 2021. "Healthcare Industry to Undergo Big Changes by 2040." *Treasury & Risk.* https://www.treasuryandrisk.com/2021/02/28/big-changes-trillions-in-savings-deloitte-makes-predictions-about-health-care-in-2040-411-24537/.

13 ***As an example*** - Miliard, M. 2021. "Kaiser Permanente Inks Multiyear Cloud Deal with Microsoft, Accenture." *Healthcare IT News.* https://www.healthcareitnews.com/news/kaiser-permanente-inks-multi-year-cloud-deal-microsoft-accenture.

13 ***The alliance with*** – Walgreens. 2021. "Walgreens Boots Alliance Makes $5.2 Billion Investment in VillageMD to Deliver Value-Based Primary Care to Communities Across America." https://news.walgreens.com/press-center/walgreens-boots-alliance-makes-52-billion-investment-in-villagemd-to-deliver-value-based-primary-care-to-communities-across-america.htm.

14 ***Digitizing many parts*** - "Goldman Sachs: Digital Revolution Can Save $300 Billion on Healthcare." 2015. *EMSWorld.* https://www.hmpgloballearningnetwork.com/site/emsworld/news/12091550/goldman-sachs-digital-revolution-can-save-300-billion-on-healthcare.

14 ***Labor and medical supply expenses*** - Muoio, D. 2022. "AHA: Federal Funds Needed to Offset 20% Per-Patient Increase in Hospital Expenses since 2019." *Fierce Healthcare.* https://www.fiercehealthcare.com/providers/aha-federal-funds-needed-offset-20-patient-increase-hospital-expenses-2019.

15 ***Approximately 80 percent of health care expenses*** – Gebreyes, K., et al. 2021. "Breaking the Cost Curve." *Modern Healthcare.* https://www.modernhealthcare.com/finance/breaking-cost-curve.

15 ***Currently, there are*** - Mather, M., P. Scommegna, and L. Kilduff. 2019. "Fact Sheet: Aging in the United States." *PRB.* https://www.prb.org/resources/fact-sheet-aging-in-the-united-states/.

16 ***With self-management approaches*** - Zhao, M., J. H. Wasfy, and J. P. Singh. 2020. "Sensor-Aided Continuous Care and Self-Management: Implications for the Post-COVID Era." *Lancet Digital Health* 2:e632–e634.

PART I: SENSORS

1: MAKING SENSE OF SENSORS

21 ***The sensory system is a web*** - Walsh, V. 2017. "Sensory Systems." *Reference Module in Neuroscience and Biobehavioral Psychology*. doi:10.1016/B978-0-12-809324-5.06867-X.

22 ***Basically, there are five*** - Vosshall, L. B., and M. Carandini. 2009. "Sensory Systems." *Curr Opin Neurobiol* 19:343–44.

23 ***Just recently, in*** - Ledford, H., and E. Callaway. 2021. "Medicine Nobel Goes to Scientists Who Discovered Biology of Senses." *Nature* 598:246.

25 ***Like an automobile*** - Münzl, M. 2018. "The Human Body as an Analogy for Automation." *Balluff Blog*. https://www.innovating-automation.blog/the-human-body-as-an-analogy-for-automation/.

26 ***Outside the human body*** - Fraden, J. 2014. *Handbook of Modern Sensors: Physics, Designs, and Applications*. New York: Springer.

27 ***The future is dependent upon*** - Merchant, F. M., G. W. Dec, and J. P. Singh. 2010. "Implantable Sensors for Heart Failure." *Circ Arrhythm Electrophysiol* 3:657–67.

27 ***Easily available biological fluids*** - Dang, W., et al. 2018. "Stretchable Wireless System for Sweat pH Monitoring." *Biosens Bioelectron* 107:192–202.

28 ***Implanted devices, which provide continuous*** - Bussooa, A., S. Neale, and J. R. Mercer. 2018. "Future of Smart Cardiovascular Implants." *Sensors (Basel)* 18:e2008.

28 ***A host of simple sensors*** - Gardner, R. S., et al. 2018. "HeartLogic Multisensor Algorithm Identifies Patients during Periods of Significantly Increased Risk of Heart Failure Events: Results from the MultiSENSE Study." *Circ Heart Fail* 11:e004669.

29 ***Empowering patients to self-manage*** - Zhao, M., J. H. Wasfy, and J. P. Singh. 2020. "Sensor-Aided Continuous Care and Self-Management: Implications for the Post-COVID Era." *Lancet Digit Health* 2:e632–e634.

2: DOC-IN-THE-BOX

33 ***When we look at the data*** - Sana, F., et al. 2020. "Wearable Devices for Ambulatory Cardiac Monitoring: JACC State-of-the-Art Review." *J Am Coll Cardiol* 75:1582–92.

33 ***PPG can gather*** - Moraes, J. L., et al. 2018. "Advances in Photoplethysmography Signal Analysis for Biomedical Applications." *Sensors (Basel)* 18:E1894.

33 ***A breathing instrument*** - Paiva, R. P., P. de Carvalho, and V. Kilintzis. 2022. *Wearable*

Sensing and Intelligent Data Analysis for Respiratory Management. Cambridge, MA: Academic Press.

34 ***Even contact-free PPG algorithms*** - Castaneda, D., et al. 2018. "A Review on Wearable Photoplethysmography Sensors and Their Potential Future Applications in Health Care." *Int J Biosens Bioelectron* 4:195–202.

35 ***Care will be automated*** - Zhao, M., J. H. Wasfy, and J. P. Singh. 2020. "Sensor-Aided Continuous Care and Self-management: Implications for the Post-COVID Era." *Lancet Digit Health* 2:e632–e634.

35 ***Research has shown*** - Sohn, K., et al. 2019. "Utility of a Smartphone Based System (cvrPhone) to Predict Short-term Arrhythmia Susceptibility." *Sci Rep* 9:14497.

35 ***The fluctuation in lung function*** - Sohn, K., et al. 2017. "A Novel Point-of-Care Smartphone Based System for Monitoring the Cardiac and Respiratory Systems." *Sci Rep* 7:44946.

35 ***The flow rate can then*** - Sohn, K., et al. 2019. "Utility of a Smartphone Based System (cvrphone) to Accurately Determine Apneic Events from Electrocardiographic Signals." *PLoS One* 14, e0217217.

36 ***Smartphones can also help*** - Bauer, M., et al. 2020. "Smartphones in Mental Health: A Critical Review of Background Issues, Current Status and Future Concerns." *Int J Bipolar Disord* 8:2.

36 ***Phone usage*** - Wacks, Y., and A. M. Weinstein. 2021. "Excessive Smartphone Use Is Associated with Health Problems in Adolescents and Young Adults." *Frontiers in Psychiatry* 12:1–7.

36 ***An app called Autism & Beyond*** - Duke Today Staff. 2015. "Duke Launches Autism Research App." https://today.duke.edu/2015/10/autismbeyond.

36 ***Compare the data*** - Wilhelm, S., et al. 2020. "Development and Pilot Testing of a Cognitive-Behavioral Therapy Digital Service for Body Dysmorphic Disorder." *Behavior Therapy* 51:15–26.

37 ***For example, Parkinson's disease*** - Zhang, T., et al. 2021. "Smartphone Applications in the Management of Parkinson's Disease in a Family Setting: An Opinion Article." *Front Neurol* 12:668953.

38 ***In patients with depression*** - Osmani, V. 2015. "Smartphones in Mental Health: Detecting Depressive and Manic Episodes." *IEEE Pervasive Computing* 14:10–13.

38 ***And diabetes*** - Liu, Q., et al. 2018. "Highly Sensitive and Wearable In2O3 Nanoribbon Transistor Biosensors with Integrated On-Chip Gate for Glucose Monitoring in Body Fluids." *ACS Nano* 12:1170–78.

39 ***Colorimetric tests from body fluids*** - Hong, J. I., and B.-Y. Chang. 2014. "Development of the Smartphone-Based Colorimetry for Multi-Analyte Sensing Arrays." *Lab Chip* 14:1725–32.

39 ***Is smart fabrics*** - Sayol, I. 2020. "Smart Fabrics, a Technology that Revolutionizes Experiences." *Ignasi Sayol*. https://ignasisayol.com/en/smart-textiles-can-be-programmed-to-monitor-things-like-biometrics-measurements-of-physical-attributes-or-behaviours-like-heart-rate-which-could-help-athletes-dieters-and-physicians-observing-pat/.

40 ***Smart socks*** - Pai, A. 2015. "Researchers Develop Pressure Sensing Socks for People with Diabetes." *MobiHealthNews*. https://www.mobihealthnews.com/43511/researchers-develop-pressure-sensing-socks-for-people-with-diabetes.

40 ***pH sensors*** - Sun, A., et al. 2017. "Smartphone-Based pH Sensor for Home Monitoring of Pulmonary Exacerbations in Cystic Fibrosis." *Sensors* 17:1245.

41 ***Tattoo sensors that can be*** - Kabiri Ameri, S., et al. 2017. "Graphene Electronic Tattoo Sensors." *ACS Nano* 11:7634–41.

41 ***Cheap, highly customizable*** - Bandodkar, A. J., W. Jia, and J. Wang. 2015. "Tattoo-Based Wearable Electrochemical Devices: A Review." *Electroanalysis* 27:562–72.

3: THE FAILING HEART, THE DYING PATIENT, AND IMPLANTABLE SENSORS

45 ***It affects more than 6.5 million*** - Jackson, S. L., et al. 2018. "National Burden of Heart Failure Events in the United States, 2006 to 2014." *Circulation: Heart Failure* 11:e004873.

45 ***This disease drains*** - Heidenreich, P. A., et al. 2018. "Forecasting the Impact of Heart Failure in the United States." *Circulation: Heart Failure* 6:606–19.

47 ***Believe it or not*** - Merchant, F. M., G. W. Dec, and J. P. Singh. 2010. "Implantable Sensors for Heart Failure." *Circ Arrhythm Electrophysiol* 3:657–67.

47 ***The beat-to-beat*** - Singh, J. P., et al. 1997. "QT Interval Dynamics and Heart Rate Variability Preceding a Case of Cardiac Arrest." *Heart* 77:375–77.

47 ***Heart rate variability*** - Singh, J. P., et al. 2000. "Association of Hyperglycemia with Reduced Heart Rate Variability (The Framingham Heart Study)." *Am J Cardiol* A86:309–12.

47 ***Heart rate variability*** - Singh, J. P., et al. 1998. "Reduced Heart Rate Variability and New-Onset Hypertension." *Hypertension* 32:293–97.

50 ***Just a change in*** - Moraes, J. L., et al. 2018. "Advances in Photoplethysmography Signal Analysis for Biomedical Applications." *Sensors (Basel)* 18:E1894.

51 ***Served to directly measure*** - Troughton, R. W., et al. 2011. "Direct Left Atrial Pressure

Monitoring in Severe Heart Failure: Long-term Sensor Performance." *J Cardiovasc Transl Res* 4:3–13.

52 ***A clinical trial called Diagnostic Outcome Trial in Heart Failure*** - van Veldhuisen, D. J., et al. 2011. "Intrathoracic Impedance Monitoring, Audible Patient Alerts, and Outcome in Patients with Heart Failure." *Circulation* 124:1719–26.

54 ***A proprietary algorithm incorporating*** - Boehmer, J. P., et al. 2017. "A Multisensor Algorithm Predicts Heart Failure Events in Patients with Implanted Devices: Results from the MultiSENSE Study." *JACC Heart Fail* 5:216–25.

54 ***Is a hormone released*** - Gardner, R. S., et al. 2018. "HeartLogic Multisensor Algorithm Identifies Patients during Periods of Significantly Increased Risk of Heart Failure Events: Results from the MultiSENSE Study." *Circ Heart Fail* 11:e004669.

56 ***For instance, there is great*** - Tsai, N.-C., and C.-Y. Sue. 2007. "Review of MEMS-Based Drug Delivery and Dosing Systems." *Sens Actuator A Phys* 134:555–64.

56 ***Development of microelectromechanical systems*** - Cobo, A., R. Sheybani, and E. Meng. 2015. "MEMS: Enabled Drug Delivery Systems." *Adv Healthc Mater* 4:969–82.

58 ***A multidisciplinary forum*** - Altman, R. K., et al. 2012. "Multidisciplinary Care of Patients Receiving Cardiac Resynchronization Therapy Is Associated with Improved Clinical Outcomes." *Eur Heart J* 33:2181–88.

4: THE SMARTWATCH ERA

63 ***The same physiological signals*** - Hajj-Boutros, G., et al. 2022. "Wrist-Worn Devices for the Measurement of Heart Rate and Energy Expenditure: A Validation Study for the Apple Watch 6, Polar Vantage V and Fitbit Sense." *Eur J Sport Sci* 1–13. doi:10.1080/17461391.2021.2023656.

64 ***I recently interviewed*** - Lubitz, S. A., et al. 2021. "Rationale and Design of a Large Population Study to Validate Software for the Assessment of Atrial Fibrillation from Data Acquired by a Consumer Tracker or Smartwatch: The Fitbit Heart Study." *Am Heart J* 238:16–26.

64 ***Apple Heart Study*** - Perez, M. V., et al. 2019. "Large-Scale Assessment of a Smartwatch to Identify Atrial Fibrillation." *N Engl J Med* 381:1909–17.

65 ***Many companies*** - Maille, B., et al. 2021. "Smartwatch Electrocardiogram and Artificial Intelligence for Assessing Cardiac-Rhythm Safety of Drug Therapy in the COVID-19 Pandemic. The QT-logs study." *Int J Cardiol* 331:333–39.

65 ***Imagine a tool like*** - Singh, J. P., et al. 2022. "Short-Term Prediction of Atrial Fibrillation from Ambulatory Monitoring ECG Using a Deep Neural Network." *Eur Heart J Digit Health* ztac014. doi:10.1093/ehjdh/ztac014.

65 ***Not everyone is a fan*** - Kowey, P. 2019. "Indeed, Dr. Packer, What Did the Apple Heart Study Achieve?" *Medpage Today.* https://www.medpagetoday.com/cardiology/arrhythmias/78932.

66 ***The ultimate guardian*** - Martellaro, J. 2018. "The Apple Watch Is Now the Intelligent Guardian of the Galaxy." *Mac Observer.* https://www.macobserver.com/columns-opinions/editorial/apple-watch-intelligent-guardian/.

66 ***The accuracy of the*** - 2019 "Apple Heart Study Identifies AFib in Small Group of Apple Watch Wearers." *American College of Cardiology.* https://www.acc.org/latest-in-cardiology/articles/apple-heart-study-acc-2019A.

67 ***One-fifth of all strokes*** - Pistoia, F., et al. 2016. "The Epidemiology of Atrial Fibrillation and Stroke." *Cardiol Clin* 34:255–68.

67 ***The well-publicized*** - Bray, H. 2021. "A Smart Watch Could Save Your Life." *Boston Globe.* https://www.bostonglobe.com/2021/08/23/business/how-smart-watch-could-save-your-life/.

68 ***Seamlessly integrated into*** - Sahu, M. L., et al. 2021. "IoT-Enabled Cloud-Based Real-Time Remote ECG Monitoring System." *J Med Eng Technol* 45:473–85.

68 ***Need for a digital*** - Haelle, T. 2021. "Wearable Fitness Trackers Could Detect COVID before You Do." *WebMD.* https://www.webmd.com/lung/news/20211130/wearable-fitness-trackers-covid.

69 ***Pick up early infections*** - Mishra, T., et al. 2020. "Pre-Symptomatic Detection of COVID-19 from Smartwatch Data." *Nat Biomed Eng* 4:1208–20.

69 ***Real-time detection of COVID-19*** - Sherburne, M. 2022. "Wearables Can Track COVID Symptoms, Other Diseases." *University of Michigan News.* https://news.umich.edu/wearables-can-track-covid-symptoms-other-diseases/.

70 ***Almost 20 percent*** - Vogels, E. A. 2020. "About One-in-Five Americans Use a Smart Watch or Fitness Tracker." *Pew Research Center.* https://www.pewresearch.org/fact-tank/2020/01/09/about-one-in-five-americans-use-a-smart-watch-or-fitness-tracker/.

5: CONTINUOUS CARE AND NOVEL SENSORS: A RECIPE FOR HEALTH

72 ***Disease that affects more than thirty million people*** - Centers for Disease Control

and Prevention. 2022. "National Diabetes Statistics Report." https://www.cdc.gov/diabetes/data/statistics-report/index.html.

73 ***Kidney failure, heart attacks*** - Mendola, N. D., et al. 2018. "Prevalence of Total, Diagnosed, and Undiagnosed Diabetes Among Adults: United States, 2013–2016." 8.

73 ***BlueStar diabetes management solutions*** - Gopisetty, D. 2019. "BlueStar App Now Integrates with CGM and Approved for Type 1 Diabetes." *diatribe.* https://diatribe.org/bluestar-app-now-integrates-cgm-and-approved-type-1-diabetes.

74 ***There are FDA-approved oral devices*** - Comstock, J. 2015. "Sleep Apnea Treatment Device with Wireless Compliance Sensor Gets FDA Nod." *MobiHealthNews.* https://www.mobihealthnews.com/44719/sleep-apnea-treatment-device-with-wireless-compliance-sensor-gets-fda-nod.

74 ***Sleep apnea*** - Bonato, R. 2013. "Introducing a Novel Micro-Recorder for the Detection of Oral Appliance Compliance: DentiTrac." *Sleep Diagnosis and Therapy* 8 (3): 12–15. https://www.aaosh.org/connect/introducing-novel-micro-recorder-detection-oral-appliance-compliance-dentitrac.

74 ***Wearable UV sensors*** - Hu, N., et al. 2020. "Wearable Bracelet Monitoring the Solar Ultraviolet Radiation for Skin Health Based on Hybrid IPN Hydrogels." *ACS Appl. Mater. Interfaces* 12:56480–490.

77 ***The synergy between*** - Kumar, S., P. Tiwari, and M. Zymbler. 2019. "Internet of Things Is a Revolutionary Approach for Future Technology Enhancement: A Review." *J Big Data* 6:111.

77 ***Create the IoT*** - Kang, M., et al. 2018. "Recent Patient Health Monitoring Platforms Incorporating Internet of Things-Enabled Smart Devices." *Int Neurourol J* 22:S76–82.

78 ***The use of alternative analytes*** - Hong, J. I., and B.-Y. Chang. 2014. "Development of the Smartphone-Based Colorimetry for Multi-Analyte Sensing Arrays." *Lab Chip* 14:1725–32.

78 ***Poor adherence*** - Viswanathan, M., et al. 2012. "Interventions to Improve Adherence to Self-Administered Medications for Chronic Diseases in the United States." *Ann Intern Med* 157:785–95.

79 ***Newer, ingestible*** - Flores, G. P., et al. 2016. "Performance, Reliability, Usability, and Safety of the ID-Cap System for Ingestion Event Monitoring in Healthy Volunteers: A Pilot Study." *Innov Clin Neurosci* 13:12–19.

79 ***Artificial tactile sensors*** - Girão, P. S., et al. 2013. "Tactile Sensors for Robotic Applications." *Measurement* 46:1257–71.

79 ***Progression of glaucoma*** - National Institute for Health and Care Excellence. 2014. "The

SENSIMED Triggerfish Contact Lens Sensor for Continuous 24-Hour Recording of Ocular Dimensional Changes in People with or at Risk of Developing Glaucoma." https://www.nice.org.uk/advice/mib14/resources/thesensimed-triggerfish-contact-lens-sensor-for-continuous-24hour-recording-of-ocular-dimensional-changes-in-people-with-or-at-risk-of-developing-glaucoma-63498984662725.

80 ***Smart contact lenses*** - Elsherif, M., et al. 2022. "Wearable Smart Contact Lenses for Continual Glucose Monitoring: A Review." *Front Med* 9:1–15.

80 ***Correlation of these*** - "Glucose Sensor: An Overview." ScienceDirect Topics. https://www.sciencedirect.com/topics/engineering/glucose-sensor.

80 ***Such as the ADAMM device*** - Rhee, H., et al. 2014. "The Development of an Automated Device for Asthma Monitoring for Adolescents: Methodologic Approach and User Acceptability." *JMIR Mhealth Uhealth* 2:e27.

80 ***iBGStar*** - Shelly, J., and S. Ferreri. 2012. "iBGStar: The 'iPhone Blood Glucose Meter.'" *Pharmacy Today* 18:28.

80 ***Other sensors in the*** - Milstein, N., and I. Gordon. 2020. "Validating Measures of Electrodermal Activity and Heart Rate Variability Derived from the Empatica E4 Utilized in Research Settings That Involve Interactive Dyadic States." *Front Behav Neurosci* 14.

81 ***This is known as blepharospasm*** - Mahmood, M., et al. 2020. "Soft Nanomembrane Sensors and Flexible Hybrid Bioelectronics for Wireless Quantification of Blepharospasm." *IEEE Transactions on Biomedical Engineering* 67:3094–3100.

82 ***When speaking with*** - Singh, J. P. 2021. "Booze Out, Coffee Okay to Outsmart AF?" *Medscape.* https://www.medscape.com/viewarticle/961993.

82 ***These are called N of 1 trials*** - Marcus, G. 2022. "N-of-1 Randomized Trials: CRAVE and I-STOP-AFib as Examples (Gregory Marcus, MD, MAS)." *Rethinking Clinical Trials.* https://rethinkingclinicaltrials.org/news/grand-rounds-may-6-n-of-1-randomized-trials-crave-and-i-stop-afib-as-examples-gregory-marcus-md-mas/ (2022).

84 ***BOAT OAR*** - Saint Luke's Health System. 2022. "Better Outcomes for Anticoagulation Treatment through Observation of Atrial Rhythm (BOAT OAR)." https://clinicaltrials.gov/ct2/show/NCT03515083.

86 ***mHealth tools*** - Olsen, E. 2021. "Welldoc's Bluestar Lands FDA Clearance for Expanded Insulin Dosing Support." *MobiHealthNews.* https://www.mobihealthnews.com/news/welldocs-bluestar-lands-fda-clearance-expanded-insulin-dosing-support.

86 ***They recently called for*** - Data Science at NIH. 2022 "NIH Fast Healthcare Interoperability Resources Initiatives." https://datascience.nih.gov/fhir-initiatives.

86 ***As innovative technology*** - Singh, J. 2020. "The Digital Divide Can Kill—Can We Bridge

It?" *Medium.* https://jagsinghmd.medium.com/the-digital-divide-can-kill-can-we-bridge-it-93b136bdaf35.

86 ***It will become*** - Singh, J. P. 2018. "Connecting Life with Devices." *JACC Clin Electrophysiol* 4:422–23.

PART II: VIRTUAL CARE

6: TELEHEALTH: FAD OR HERE TO STAY?

91 ***Nearly $200 billion*** - Global Market Insights. 2020. "Telemedicine Market Expected to Hit $175 Billion by 2026." *Healthcare Facilities Today.* https://www.healthcarefacilitiestoday.com/posts/Telemedicine-Market-Expected-to-Hit-175-Billion-by-2026--24943.

91 ***It gave new life to this mode*** - Wosik, J., et al. 2020. "Telehealth Transformation: COVID-19 and the Rise of Virtual Care." *J Am Med Inform Assoc* 27:957–62.

91 ***Virtual care was here*** - Singh, J. 2020. "Virtual Care: Fad or Here to Stay?" *Medium.* https://jagsinghmd.medium.com/virtual-care-fad-or-here-to-stay-a2afb2ddea50.

91 ***In a separate survey*** - The COVID-19 Healthcare Coalition Telehealth Impact Study Work Group. 2021. "Telehealth Impact: Patient Survey Analysis." *COVID-19 Healthcare Coalition.* https://c19hcc.org/telehealth/patient-survey-analysis/.

91 ***The rise in telehealth*** - Polinski, J. M., et al. 2016. "Patients' Satisfaction with and Preference for Telehealth Visits." *J Gen Intern Med* 31:269–75.

91 ***Acceptance and adoption*** - Andrews, E., et al. 2020. "Satisfaction with the Use of Telehealth during COVID-19: An integrative review." *International Journal of Nursing Studies Advances* 2, 100008.

92 ***The funding for digital health*** - Krasniansky, A., et al. 2022. "2021 Year-End Digital Health Funding: Seismic Shifts beneath the Surface." Rock Health. https://rockhealth.com/insights/2021-year-end-digital-health-funding-seismic-shifts-beneath-the-surface/.

93 ***Telehealth, with its virtual interactive*** - Global Market Insights Inc. 2021. "Telemedicine Market Size & Share, Growth Outlook 2021–2027." https://www.gminsights.com/industry-analysis/telemedicine-market.

93 ***Goldman Sachs estimates that*** - 2015. "Goldman Sachs: Digital Revolution Can Save $300 Billion on Healthcare." *EMSWorld.* https://www.hmpgloballearningnetwork.com/site/emsworld/news/12091550/goldman-sachs-digital-revolution-can-save-300-billion-on-healthcare.

93 ***A professor from*** - Groysberg, B., and K. C. Baden. 2020. "The COVID Two-Step for Leaders: Protect and Pivot." *HBS Working Knowledge.* http://hbswk.hbs.edu/item/the-covid-two-step-for-leaders-protect-and-pivot.

95 ***Concomitant increase in*** - Lee, N. T., J. Karsten, and J. Roberts. 2020. "Removing Regulatory Barriers to Telehealth before and after COVID-19." Brookings Foundation 24.

95 ***Will be scaled back*** - Advisory Board. 2022. "Is the Pandemic-Era Telehealth Boom Reversing?" https://www.advisory.com/Daily-Briefing/2022/01/05/telehealth.

96 ***Within the state border*** - Blackman, K. 2016. "Telehealth and Licensing Interstate Providers." *National Conference of State Legislatures.* https://www.ncsl.org/research/health/telehealth-and-licensing-interstate-providers.aspx.

96 ***Quantitative and actionable data*** - Holko, M., et al. 2022. "Wearable Fitness Tracker Use in Federally Qualified Health Center Patients: Strategies to Improve the Health of All of Us Using Digital Health Devices." *NPJ Digit Med* 5:53.

97 ***The McKinsey Global Institute has estimated*** - *The Future of Work after COVID-19.* New York: McKinsey Global.

99 ***The tele-visit does not*** - Rosenthal, E. 2021. "Opinion: Telemedicine Is a Tool. Not a Replacement for Your Doctor's Touch." *New York Times.* www.nytimes.com/2021/04/29/opinion/virtual-remote-medicine-covid.html.

100 ***We have already begun*** - Zhao, M., et al. 2021. "Virtual Multidisciplinary Care for Heart Failure Patients with Cardiac Resynchronization Therapy Devices during the Coronavirus Disease 2019 Pandemic." *Int J Cardiol Heart Vasc* 34:100811.

100 ***All I need to do is*** - Rasmussen, P. 2022. LinkedIn. https://www.linkedin.com/feed/update/urn:li:activity:6939951602556424193/.

102 ***Large distances across*** - Kye, B., et al. 2021. "Educational Applications of Metaverse: Possibilities and Limitations." *J Educ Eval Health Prof* 18:1–13.

102 ***Add to this sensor-derived data*** - Skalidis, I., O. Muller, and S. Fournier. 2022. "CardioVerse: The Cardiovascular Medicine in the Era of Metaverse." *Trends in Cardiovascular Medicine.* doi:10.1016/j.tcm.2022.05.004.

102 ***Treating situational phobias*** - Ifdil, I., et al. 2022. "Virtual Reality in Metaverse for Future Mental Health-Helping Profession: An Alternative Solution to the Mental Health Challenges of the COVID-19 Pandemic." *J Public Health (Oxf)* 1–2. doi:10.1093/pubmed/fdac049.

7: ARE WE BREAKING THE BANK?

105 ***Signs of a quick rewind*** - Advisory Board. 2022. "Is the Pandemic-Era Telehealth Boom Reversing?" https://www.advisory.com/Daily-Briefing/2022/01/05/telehealth.

106 ***Dermatology has made some*** - American Academy of Dermatoloty Association. 2022. "Telemedicine: Overview." https://www.aad.org/public/fad/telemedicine.

106 ***Many AI algorithms*** - Woźniacka, A., S. Patrzyk, and M. Mikołajczyk. 2021. "Artificial Intelligence in Medicine and Dermatology." *Postepy Dermatol Alergol* 38:948–52.

107 ***Even rheumatology*** - American College of Rheumatology Position Statement (2020). https://www.rheumatology.org/Portals/0/Files/Telemedicine-Position-Statement.pdf.

107 ***One such program*** - Scirica, B. M., et al. 2021. "Digital Care Transformation." *Circulation* 143:507–9.

108 ***App-based cognitive*** - Wilhelm, S., et al. 2020. "Development and Pilot Testing of a Cognitive-Behavioral Therapy Digital Service for Body Dysmorphic Disorder." *Behavior Therapy* 51:15–26.

108 ***Tele-neurology is one*** - Ali, F., et al. 2020. "Role of Artificial Intelligence in TeleStroke: An Overview." *Front Neurosci* 11.

109 ***And the 6G*** - Kranz, G. and G. Christensen. 2022. "What Is 6G & When Is It Available?" *SearchNetworking*. https://www.techtarget.com/searchnetworking/definition/6G.

110 ***Lower price per virtual*** - Kopf, M. 2022. "The Cost of a Telehealth Visit." *K Health*. https://khealth.com/learn/healthcare/telehealth-visit-cost/.

110 ***Intermountain Healthcare's telehealth program*** - Cheney, C. 2018. "How Intermountain Saved $1.2M with Neonatal Telehealth Program." *HealthLeaders Media*. https://www.healthleadersmedia.com/clinical-care/how-intermountain-saved-12m-neonatal-telehealth-program.

110 ***Newborn*** - Albritton, J., et al. 2018. "The Effect of a Newborn Telehealth Program on Transfers Avoided: A Multiple-Baseline Study." *Health Affairs* 37:1990–96.

111 ***Connect with a digital community*** - Mirsky, J. B., and A. N. Thorndike. 2021. "Virtual Group Visits: Hope for Improving Chronic Disease Management in Primary Care during and after the COVID-19 Pandemic." *Am J Health Promot* 35:904–7.

111 ***One of the biggest drivers*** - Reed, T. 2019. "Report: US Economic Burden of Chronic Diseases Tops $3.8 Trillion—and Expected to Double." *Fierce Healthcare*. https://www.fiercehealthcare.com/hospitals-health-systems/fitch-rain (2019).

111 ***And the CDC has reported*** - Health and Economic Costs of Chronic Diseases https://www.cdc.gov/chronicdisease/about/costs/index.htm (2022).

8: THE DEEPENING DIVIDE

114 ***Telemonitoring platforms*** - Gokalp, H., et al. 2018. "Integrated Telehealth and Telecare for Monitoring Frail Elderly with Chronic Disease." *Telemed J E Health* AU24:940–57.

115 ***Unless automated*** - Ikram, U., et al. 2020. "4 Strategies to Make Telehealth Work for Elderly Patients." *HarvBus Rev.* https://hbr.org/2020/11/4-strategies-to-make-telehealth-work-for-elderly-patients.

116 ***Sensor sophistication*** - Holko, M., et al. 2022. "Wearable Fitness Tracker Use in Federally Qualified Health Center Patients: Strategies to Improve the Health of All of Us Using Digital Health Devices." *NPJ Digit Med* 5:53.

117 ***Our research work*** - Brown, K. J., et al. 2021. "Social Determinants of Telemedicine Utilization in Ambulatory Cardiovascular Patients during the COVID-19 Pandemic." *Eur Heart J - Digital Health* 2:244–53.

117 ***The structural discrepancies*** - Singh, J. 2020. "The Digital Divide Can Kill—Can We Bridge it?" *Medium.* https://jagsinghmd.medium.com/the-digital-divide-can-kill-can-we-bridge-it-93b136bdaf35.

117 ***Individuals from these marginalized*** - Singh, A., et al. 2020. "The Evolving Face of Cardiovascular Care in the Peri-pandemic Era." *Harvard Health Policy Rev.* http://www.hhpronline.org/articles/2020/11/16/the-evolving-face-of-cardiovascular-care-in-the-peri-pandemic-era.

118 ***With continuous environmental exposure*** - Centers for Disease Control and Prevention. 2020. "Risk for COVID-19 Infection, Hospitalization, and Death by Race/Ethnicity." https://www.cdc.gov/coronavirus/2019-ncov/covid-data/investigations-discovery/hospitalization-death-by-race-ethnicity.html.

118 ***And now, the digital divide*** - Philbin, M. M., et al. 2019. "Health Disparities and the Digital Divide: The Relationship between Communication Inequalities and Quality of Life among Women in a Nationwide Prospective Cohort Study in the United States." *J Health Commun* 24:405–12.

118 ***But also inner-city and urban areas*** - Eruchalu, C. N., et al. 2021. "The Expanding Digital Divide: Digital Health Access Inequities during the COVID-19 Pandemic in New York City." *J Urban Health* 98:183–86.

118 ***Has gained notoriety*** - Litchfield, I., D. Shukla, and S. Greenfield. 2021. "Impact of COVID-19 on the Digital Divide: A Rapid Review." *BMJ Open* 11:e053440.

119 ***Internet access should be*** - Sun, N., et al. 2020. "Human Rights and Digital Health Technologies." *Health Hum Rights* 22:21–32.

119 ***The Healthcare Connect Fund Program aims*** - "Healthcare Connect Fund Program." *Universal Service Administrative Company.* https://www.usac.org/rural-health-care/healthcare-connect-fund-program/.

119 ***Connected Care Pilot Program*** - Federal Communications Commission. 2020. "Connected Care Pilot Program." https://www.fcc.gov/wireline-competition/telecommunications-access-policy-division/connected-care-pilot-program.

120 ***More than 85 percent*** - O'Dea, S. 2022. "Smartphones in the US: Statistics & Facts." *Statista.* https://www.statista.com/topics/2711/us-smartphone-market/.

120 ***Distribution of free*** - "Mass General Brigham Launches New Digital Health Initiatives." Mass General Brigham. https://www.massgeneralbrigham.org/newsroom/press-releases/mass-general-brigham-launches-new-digital-health-initiatives.

121 ***Care crosses national*** - World Health Organization. 2022. "Digital Health." https://www.who.int/health-topics/digital-health.

122 ***Enmeshed in war*** - GlobalData Thematic Research. 2022. "The Telemedicine Community Has Rallied to Provide Support to Patients in Ukraine." *Pharmaceutical Technology.* https://www.pharmaceutical-technology.com/comment/telemedicine-community-support-ukraine/.

9: DIGITAL PRIVACY—AN OXYMORON?

124 ***And then the breach happened*** - Stockley, M. 2018. "150 Million MyFitnessPal Accounts Compromised—Here's What to Do." *Naked Security.* https://nakedsecurity.sophos.com/2018/03/30/150-million-myfitnesspal-accounts-compromised-heres-what-to-do/.

124 ***The hackers had*** - Newcomb, A. 2019. "Hacked MyFitnessPal Data Goes on Sale on the Dark Web—One Year after the Breach." *Fortune.* https://fortune.com/2019/02/14/hacked-myfitnesspal-data-sale-dark-web-one-year-breach/.

124 ***And then there is a library*** - Wicklund, E. 2018. "UK's NHS Aims to Build a Library of Reliable Mobile Health Apps." *mHealthIntelligence.* https://mhealthintelligence.com/news/uks-nhs-aims-to-build-a-library-of-reliable-mobile-health-apps.

124 ***Approximately 20 percent of them*** - Gallagher, L. 2015. "Information Handling by Some Health Apps Not as Secure as It Should Be." *Imperial News.* https://www.imperial.ac.uk/news/167866/information-handling-some-health-apps-secure/.

125 ***The PEW Research Center has suggested*** - Pew Research Center. 2022. "Texting." https://www.pewresearch.org/topic/internet-technology/platforms-services/mobile/texting/.

126 ***Kick Butts is a text-based tobacco*** - Kick Butts Program. 2020. "Kick Butts Program, Become a Non-Smoker Again." https://kickbuttsprogram.com/.

126 ***These have been shown to*** - 2016. Patel, M.S. "Patients Had Shorter Hospital Stays When Their Care Providers Used Secure Text Messaging to Improve Communication, Penn Study Finds." *Penn Medicine News.* https://www.pennmedicine.org/news/news-releases/2016/april/patients-had-shorter-hospital.

126 ***And ER visits*** - Patel, M. S., et al. 2016. "Change In Length of Stay and Readmissions among Hospitalized Medical Patients after Inpatient Medicine Service Adoption of Mobile Secure Text Messaging." *J Gen Intern Med* 31:863–70.

126 ***Disease management platforms*** - Noonan, P. 2022. "Using Personalized Text Messages to Improve Heart Failure Hospital Readmission Rates." *J Card Fail* 28:S50.

127 ***This is exemplified by the class-action*** - Eadicicco, L. 2016. "4 Things to Know about the Fitbit Accuracy Lawsuit." *Time.*

127 ***Underestimating the heart rate by approximately*** - Mole, B. 2016. "Lawsuit Claims Fitbit Devices Dangerously Underestimate Heart Rate." *Ars Technica.* https://arstechnica.com/tech-policy/2016/01/lawsuit-claims-fitbit-devices-dangerously-underestimate-heart-rate/.

127 ***Precertification pilot program*** - US Food & Drug Administration. 2022. "Digital Health Software Precertification (Pre-Cert) Pilot Program." https://www.fda.gov/medical-devices/digital-health-center-excellence/digital-health-software-precertification-pre-cert-program.

127 ***Cyberattacks that could*** - Khan, S. I., and A. S. L. Haque. 2016. "Digital Health Data: A Comprehensive Review of Privacy and Security Risks and Some Recommendations." *Comp Sci J Moldova* 24, no. 2 (71): 273–92.

128 ***Regulatory bindings*** - Bari, L. and D. P. O'Neill. 2019. "Rethinking Patient Data Privacy in the Era of Digital Health." *Health Affairs Forefront.* https://www.healthaffairs.org/do/10.1377/forefront.20191210.216658/full/.

PART III: ARTIFICIAL INTELLIGENCE

10: DEMYSTIFYING AI

132 ***Narrow forms of AI*** - Singh, J. P. 2019. "It Is Time for Us to Get Artificially Intelligent!" *JACC Clin Electrophysiol* 5:263–65.

132 ***Back in the 1950s*** - Turing, A. M. 1950. "Computing Machinery and Intelligence." *Mind* 59:433–60.

133 ***More recently, Amazon*** - Amazon Web Services. 2022. "What Is Artificial Intelligence?" https://aws.amazon.com/machine-learning/what-is-ai/.

133 ***The Electronic Numerical Integrator and Computer (ENIAC)*** - History Computer Staff. 2021. "ENIAC Computer- Everything You Need To Know." *History Computer.* https://history-computer.com/eniac-computer-guide/.

134 ***Machine learning*** - Johnson, K. W., et al. 2018. "Artificial Intelligence in Cardiology." *J Am Coll Cardiology* : AU71:2668–79.

136 ***Incorporation of AI into*** - Ahuja, A. S. 2019. "The Impact of Artificial Intelligence in Medicine on the Future Role of the Physician." *PeerJ* 7:e7702.

137 ***One such form of AI*** - Sadhamanus. 2020. "Counterfactual vs Contrastive Explanations in Artificial Intelligence." *Medium.* https://towardsdatascience.com/counterfactual-vs-contrastive-explanations-in-artificial-intelligence-e67a9cfc7e4e.

138 ***General-purpose technology*** - Global X Research Team. 2021. "Q&A with Erik Brynjolfsson on Disruptive Technology and the Digital Economy." *Global X ETFs.* https://www.globalxetfs.com/qa-with-erik-brynjolfsson-on-disruptive-technology-and-the-digital-economy/.

138 ***And industry analysis*** - "Artificial Intelligence (AI) in Healthcare Market Size Report, 2025." https://www.millioninsights.com.

138 ***That seven health care companies*** - Drees, J. 2020. "7 of Healthcare's Most Promising AI Companies from *Forbes*' 2020 List." *Becker's Health IT.* https://www.beckershospitalreview.com/healthcare-information-technology/7-of-healthcare-s-most-promising-ai-companies-from-forbes-2020-list.html?oly_enc_id=4824E4640690F6I.

11: CREATING THE AI CULTURE

143 ***Diagnosis of diabetic retinopathy*** - Abràmoff, M. D., et al. 2018. "Pivotal Trial of an Autonomous AI-Based Diagnostic System for Detection of Diabetic Retinopathy in Primary Care Offices." *npj Digital Med* 1:1–8.

143 ***Risk-categorize patients*** - Lee, J.-T., et al. 2021. "Prediction of Hospitalization Using Artificial Intelligence for Urgent Patients in the Emergency Department." *Sci Rep* 11:19472.

144 ***In children with autism*** - Kennedy, S. 2022. "AI Device May Help Diagnose Children's Autism in Primary Care Settings." *HealthITAnalytics.* https://healthitanalytics.com/news/ai-device-may-help-diagnose-childrens-autism-in-primary-care-settings.

144 ***An AI vendor*** - Korosec, K. 2021. "Emotion-Detection Software Startup Affectiva Ac-

quired for $73.5M." *TechCrunch.* https://social.techcrunch.com/2021/05/25/emotion-detection-software-startup-affectiva-acquired-for-73-5m/.

144 ***Cognitive decline via headshots*** - Umeda-Kameyama, Y., et al. 2021. "Screening of Alzheimer's Disease by Facial Complexion Using Artificial Intelligence." *Aging* 13:1765–72.

145 ***AI will help diagnose depression*** - Williams, I. K. 2022. "Can A.I.-Driven Voice Analysis Help Identify Mental Disorders?" *New York Times.* https://www.nytimes.com/2022/04/05/technology/ai-voice-analysis-mental-health.html.

145 ***Can AI help*** - Wooldridge, S. 2021. "Need to Pick a Doctor? Trust the AI, Study Says." *BenefitsPRO.* https://www.benefitspro.com/2021/01/06/need-to-pick-a-doctor-trust-the-ai-study-says/.

145 ***Pairing of EMRs and AI*** - Tang, A. H. 2020. "Combining AI and Electronic Health Records as a New Way to Pair Patients and Caregivers." *AIMed.* https://ai-med.io/ai-in-medicine/combining-ai-and-electronic-health-records-as-a-new-way-to-pair-patients-and-caregivers/.

146 ***Free online tools such as*** - "Chester the AI Radiology Assistant (V3)." 2019. *Machine Learning and Medicine Lab.* https://mlmed.org/tools/xray/.

146 ***Scalable across countries*** - Borkowski, A. A., et al. 2020. "Using Artificial Intelligence for COVID-19 Chest X-ray Diagnosis." *Fed Pract* 37:398–404.

146 ***Infervision's deep learning*** - "FDA Green-lights Infervision's Deep Learning Tool for Segmenting Lung CT Scans." 2020. *Legacy MedSearch.* https://legacymedsearch.com/fda-green-lights-infervisions-deep-learning-tool-for-segmenting-lung-ct-scans/.

148 ***ASCO is working on this*** - American Society of Clinical Oncology. 2022. "ASCO CancerLinQ." https://www.cancerlinq.org/.

148 ***Watson for Oncology*** - Jie, Z., Z. Zhiying, and L. Li. 2021. "A Meta-Analysis of Watson for Oncology in Clinical Application." *Sci Rep* 11:5792.

149 ***The data in cancer was*** - Konam, S. 2022. "Where Did IBM Go Wrong with Watson Health?" *Quartz.* https://qz.com/2129025/where-did-ibm-go-wrong-with-watson-health/.

149 ***Messy and filled with gaps*** - Goodwins, R. 2022. "Machine Learning the Hard Way: Watson's Fatal Misdiagnosis." *The Register.* https://www.theregister.com/2022/01/31/machine_learning_the_hard_way/.

149 ***To highlight this point*** - Yao, S., et al. 2020. "Real World Study for the Concordance between IBM Watson for Oncology and Clinical Practice in Advanced Non-Small Cell Lung Cancer Patients at a Lung Cancer Center in China." *Thorac Cancer* 11:1265–70.

149 ***The team-based approach*** - Kim, M.-S., et al. 2020. "Artificial Intelligence and Lung

Cancer Treatment Decision: Agreement with Recommendation of Multidisciplinary Tumor Board." *Transl Lung Cancer Res* 9:507–14.

151 ***Many of these toxic effects*** - Savage, N. 2021. "Tapping Into the Drug Discovery Potential of AI." *Biopharma Dealmakers.* doi:10.1038/d43747-021-00045-7.

151 ***AI might help solve*** - Staszak, M., et al. 2022. "Machine Learning in Drug Design: Use of Artificial Intelligence to Explore the Chemical Structure–Biological Activity Relationship." *Wires Comput Mol Sci* 12:e1568.

151 ***Recent work from*** - Mamoshina, P., A. Bueno-Orovio, and B. Rodriguez. 2020. "Dual Transcriptomic and Molecular Machine Learning Predicts all Major Clinical Forms of Drug Cardiotoxicity." *Front Pharmacol* 11:639.

152 ***More recently, there are scientists*** - Laubenbacher, R., et al. 2022. "Building Digital Twins of the Human Immune System: Toward a Roadmap." *npj Digit Med* 5:1–5.

152 ***There are several other arenas*** - Reed, J. 2020. "FDA Uses AI/ML for Drug Safety Predictions." *Linguamatics.* https://www.linguamatics.com/blog/fda-uses-aiml-drug-safety-predictions.

152 ***Two recent recall examples*** - Food & Drug Administration. 2021. "FDA Updates and Press Announcements on Angiotensin II Receptor Blocker (ARB) Recalls (Valsartan, Losartan, and Irbesartan)." https://www.fda.gov/drugs/drug-safety-and-availability/fda-updates-and-press-announcements-angiotensin-ii-receptor-blocker-arb-recalls-valsartan-losartan.

152 ***Metformin for diabetes*** - Walter, M. 2022. "FDA Announces a New Recall for Extended-Release Metformin Due to Contamination." *Cardiovascular Business.* https://www.cardiovascularbusiness.com/topics/clinical/heart-health/fda-announces-new-recall-extended-release-metformin-due-contamination.

153 ***Predictive models need*** - Walborn, A., et al. 2020. "Development of an Algorithm to Predict Mortality in Patients with Sepsis and Coagulopathy." *Clin Appl Thromb Hemost* 26:1–10.

154 ***Algorithms deteriorate*** - Cooper, P. B., et al. 2021. "Implementation of an Automated Sepsis Screening Tool in a Community Hospital Setting." *J Nurs Care Qual* 36:132–36.

154 ***Sepsis-prediction models*** - Persson, I., et al. 2021. "A Machine Learning Sepsis Prediction Algorithm for Intended Intensive Care Unit Use (NAVOY Sepsis): Proof-of-Concept Study." *JMIR Form Res* 5:e28000.

154 ***Or the colossal failure*** - Lazer, D., and R. Kennedy. 2015. "What We Can Learn from the Epic Failure of Google Flu Trends." *WIRED.* https://www.wired.com/2015/10/can-learn-epic-failure-google-flu-trends/.

154 ***The pandemic nevertheless*** - Ericsson Group. 2021. "Ericsson and Partners' AI and Live Network Data Offer Reliable 14-Day COVID-19 Admissions Forecast." https://www.ericsson.com/en/news/3/2021/ai-and-live-network-data-offer-reliable-14-day-covid-19-admissions-forecast.

12: LAZY, STUPID, BIASED, OR SMARTER?

155 ***Discovery of the risk factors*** - *Framingham Heart Study.* https://www.framingham-heartstudy.org/.

157 ***IBM has developed*** - Thomas, R., and F. T. O'Reilly. 2019. *The AI Ladder. Demystifying AI Challenges.* Sebastopol, CA: O'Reilly Media.

157 ***Big Data*** - Ghose, S. 2015. "Continuous Healthcare: Big Data and the Future of Medicine." *VentureBeat.* https://venturebeat.com/2015/06/21/continuous-healthcare-big-data-and-the-future-of-medicine/.

159 ***Getting data on providers*** - Song, Z., et al. 2022. "Physician Practice Pattern Variations in Common Clinical Scenarios within 5 US Metropolitan Areas." *JAMA Health Forum* 3:e214698.

159 ***Routine surveillance*** - Fraiman, J., et al. 2022. "An Estimate of the US Rate of Overuse of Screening Colonoscopy: A Systematic Review." *J Gen Intern Med* 37:1754–62.

160 ***Data science methods*** - Savova, G. K., et al. 2019. "Use of Natural Language Processing to Extract Clinical Cancer Phenotypes from Electronic Medical Records." *Cancer Research* 79:5463–70.

161 ***Extraction of information*** - Thomas, A. A., et al. 2014. "Extracting Data from Electronic Medical Records: Validation of a Natural Language Processing Program to Assess Prostate Biopsy Results." *World J Urol* 32:99–103.

163 ***This creates a dependency*** - Bishop, J. M. 2021. "Artificial Intelligence Is Stupid and Causal Reasoning Will Not Fix It." *Front Psychol* 11:513474.

164 ***The incessant data*** - Kumar, S., P. Tiwari, and M. Zymbler, M. 2019. "Internet of Things Is a Revolutionary Approach for Future Technology Enhancement: A Review." *J Big Data* 6:111.

165 ***Acceptance of AI*** - Kahn, J. 2022. "What's Wrong with 'Explainable AI.'" *Fortune.* https://fortune.com/2022/03/22/ai-explainable-radiology-medicine-crisis-eye-on-ai/.

166 ***Noninclusive and thereby*** - Daneshjou, R., et al. 2021. "Lack of Transparency and Potential Bias in Artificial Intelligence Data Sets and Algorithms: A Scoping Review." *JAMA Dermatol* 157:1362–69.

166 ***The algorithm worked*** - Haenssle, H. A., et al. 2018. "Man against Machine: Diagnostic Performance of a Deep Learning Convolutional Neural Network for Dermoscopic Melanoma Recognition in Comparison to 58 Dermatologists." *Ann Oncol* 29:1836–42.

166 ***Photographs of skin lesions*** - European Society for Medical Oncology. "Man against Machine: AI Is Better than Dermatologists at Diagnosing Skin Cancer." *ScienceDaily.* https://www.sciencedaily.com/releases/2018/05/180528190839.htm.

166 ***This exemplifies that*** - Hekler, A., et al. 2019. "Superior Skin Cancer Classification by the Combination of Human and Artificial Intelligence." *Eur J Cancer* AU120:114–21.

166 ***Not diverse enough*** - Langlotz, C., A. Kaushal, and R. Altman. 2020. "Health Care AI Systems Are Biased." *Scientific American.* https://www.scientificamerican.com/article/health-care-ai-systems-are-biased/.

166 ***Bias can find its way*** - Parikh, R. B., S. Teeple, and A. S. Navathe. 2019. "Addressing Bias in Artificial Intelligence in Health Care." *JAMA* 322:2377–78.

167 ***We need technology*** - Kumar, S., N. Setia, and A. Mahmood. 2021. "Identify and Remove Bias from AI Models." *IBM Developer.* https://developer.ibm.com/patterns/identify-and-remove-bias-from-ai-models/.

167 ***Personal prejudices*** - Hardesty, L. 2018. "Study Finds Gender and Skin-Type Bias in Commercial Artificial-Intelligence Systems." *MIT News.* https://news.mit.edu/2018/study-finds-gender-skin-type-bias-artificial-intelligence-systems-0212.

168 ***Data scientists*** - Walch, K. 2021. "How to Detect Bias in Existing AI Algorithms." *SearchEnterpriseAI.* https://www.techtarget.com/searchenterpriseai/feature/How-to-detect-bias-in-existing-AI-algorithms.

168 ***Google recently released*** - "Using the What-If Tool." *Google Cloud.* https://cloud.google.com/ai-platform/prediction/docs/using-what-if-tool.

13: PREDICTING AND PREVENTING DEATH

173 ***The best time-tested*** - Goldenberg, I., et al. 2008. "Risk Stratification for Primary Implantation of a Cardioverter-Defibrillator in Patients with Ischemic Left Ventricular Dysfunction." *J Am Coll Cardiol* 51:288–96.

173 ***Many of us*** - Singh, J. P., et al. 2005. "Factors Influencing Appropriate Firing of the Implanted Defibrillator for Ventricular Tachycardia/Fibrillation: Findings from the Multicenter Automatic Defibrillator Implantation Trial II (MADIT-II)." *J Am Coll Cardiol* 46:1712–20.

174 ***A recent study from Sweden*** - Ahmad, T., et al. 2018. "Machine Learning Methods Improve Prognostication, Identify Clinically Distinct Phenotypes, and Detect Heterogeneity in Response to Therapy in a Large Cohort of Heart Failure Patients." *J Am Heart Assoc* 7:e008081.

174 ***Will be able to ensnare diseases*** - Cedars-Sinai Medical Center. 2022. "AI May Detect Earliest Signs of Pancreatic Cancer." *ScienceDaily*. https://www.sciencedaily.com/releases/2022/04/220426153718.htm.

175 ***Risk factors for heart disease*** - Wilson, P. W. F., et al. 1998. "Prediction of Coronary Heart Disease Using Risk Factor Categories." *Circulation* 97:1837–47.

176 ***Our understanding of genetics*** - Elliott, J., et al. 2020. "Predictive Accuracy of a Polygenic Risk Score–Enhanced Prediction Model vs a Clinical Risk Score for Coronary Artery Disease." *JAMA* 323:636–45.

177 ***This has been further substantiated*** - Findlay, S. G., et al. 2020. "A Comparison of Cardiovascular Risk Scores in Native and Migrant South Asian Populations." *SSM Population Health* 11:100594.

177 ***Summated electrical signal*** - Attia, Z. I., et al. 2021. "Application of Artificial Intelligence to the Electrocardiogram." *Eur Heart J* 42:4717–30.

177 ***These insights from a*** - Harmon, D. M., Z. Attia, and P. A. Friedman. 2022. "Current and Future Implications of the Artificial Intelligence Electrocardiogram: The Transformation of Healthcare and Attendant Research Opportunities." *Cardiovasc Res* 118:e23–e25.

178 ***Beyond risk prediction*** - Sevakula, R. K., et al. 2020. "State-of-the-Art Machine Learning Techniques Aiming to Improve Patient Outcomes Pertaining to the Cardiovascular System." *J Am Heart Assoc* 9:e013924.

178 ***AI does statistically better*** - Weng, S. F., et al. 2017. "Can Machine-Learning Improve Cardiovascular Risk Prediction Using Routine Clinical Data?" *PLoS One* 12:e0174944.

178 ***Such as the QT interval*** - Maille, B., et al. 2021. "Smartwatch Electrocardiogram and Artificial Intelligence for Assessing Cardiac-Rhythm Safety of Drug Therapy in the COVID-19 Pandemic. The QT-logs study." *Int J Cardiol* 331:333–39.

178 ***And read echocardiograms*** - Alsharqi, M., et al. 2018. "Artificial Intelligence and Echocardiography." *Echo Res Pract* 5:R115–R125.

179 ***Even hemodynamic support systems*** - Diagnostic and Interventional Cardiology. 2020. "FDA Clears Data Streaming from the Impella Console to Allow Use of Artificial Intelligence Algorithms." http://www.dicardiology.com/content/fda-clears-data-streaming-impella-console-allow-use-artificial-intelligence-algorithms.

179 ***Treatment of devastating neurological*** - Saha, S., et al. 2021. "Progress in Brain Computer Interface: Challenges and Opportunities." *Front Syst Neurosci* 15:1–20.

180 ***Recent FDA clearance*** - Hale, C. 2020. "FDA Clears RapidAI's Occlusion-Spotting Stroke Software for CT Scans." *Fierce Biotech.* https://www.fiercebiotech.com/medtech/fda-clears-rapidai-s-occlusion-spotting-stroke-software-for-ct-scans.

180 ***A recent AI algorithm*** - Nimri, R., et al. 2020. "Insulin Dose Optimization Using an Automated Artificial Intelligence-Based Decision Support System in Youths with Type 1 Diabetes." *Nat Med* 26:1380–84.

180 ***Another exciting*** - Institute, N. E. 2022. "Using AI to Cure Blinding Eye Diseases." *SciTechDaily.* https://scitechdaily.com/using-ai-to-cure-blinding-eye-diseases/.

180 ***The human retina*** - Ortolan, D., et al. 2022. "Single-Cell-Resolution Map of Human Retinal Pigment Epithelium Helps Discover Subpopulations with Differential Disease Sensitivity." *Proc Natl Acad Sci USA* 119:e2117553119.

180 ***Differentiation of stem cells*** - Walter, M. 2020. "A Breakthrough in Treating Blindness: AI Helps Scientists Grow Artificial Retinal Tissue." *HealthExec.* https://healthexec.com/topics/precision-medicine/ai-scientists-artificial-retinal-tissue-blindness.

181 ***Integration of computer vision*** - Babich, N. 2020. "What Is Computer Vision & How Does It Work?" *Adobe XD Ideas.* https://xd.adobe.com/ideas/principles/emerging-technology/what-is-computer-vision-how-does-it-work/.

14: FIXES, FAILURES, AND THE FUTURE

183 ***Using AI in this*** - Weisberg, E. M., L. C. Chu, and E. K. Fishman. 2020. "The First Use of Artificial Intelligence (AI) in the ER: Triage Not Diagnosis." *Emerg Radiol* 27:361–66.

185 ***Symptom checkers*** - Isabel Healthcare. 2022. "Isabel—the Symptom Checker Doctors Use and Trust." https://symptomchecker.isabelhealthcare.com.

185 ***A smart exam platform*** - Bright.md. 2022. "Bright.md—Asynchronous Virtual Care for the Moment and the Future." https://bright.md/.

186 ***Continuous ER flow monitoring*** - Aidoc. 2020. "Emergency Room Triage With AI." https://www.aidoc.com/blog/emergency-room-triage-with-ai/.

187 ***This black-box effect*** - Savage, N. 2022. "Breaking into the Black Box of Artificial Intelligence." *Nature.* doi:10.1038/d41586-022-00858-1.

188 ***Within the field of radiology*** - Baselli, G., M. Codari, and F. Sardanelli. 2020. "Opening the Black Box of Machine Learning in Radiology: Can the Proximity of Annotated Cases Be a Way?" *Eur Radiol Exp* 4:30.

188 ***There is a projected*** - 2019. "Forbes Insights: AI and Healthcare: A Giant Opportunity." *Forbes.* https://www.forbes.com/sites/insights-intelai/2019/02/11/ai-and-healthcare-a-giant-opportunity/.

190 ***Miss Korea pageant created*** - 2013. "Korean Beauty Pageant Contestants All Look Strikingly Similar, Commenters Find." *HuffPost.* https://www.huffpost.com/entry/miss-korea-contestants-2013-photos_n_3157026.

191 ***In the post-pandemic world*** - Allam, Z. 2020. "The Rise of Machine Intelligence in the COVID-19 Pandemic and Its Impact on Health Policy." *Surveying the Covid-19 Pandemic and Its Implications* 89–96. doi:10.1016/B978-0-12-824313-8.00006-1.

191 ***Natural language processing helps*** - Genç, Ö. 2019. "The Basics of NLP and Real Time Sentiment Analysis with Open Source Tools." *Medium.* https://towardsdatascience.com/real-time-sentiment-analysis-on-social-media-with-open-source-tools-f864ca239afe.

191 ***Using a vulnerability index*** - DeCaprio, D., et al. 2020. "Building a COVID-19 Vulnerability Index." *J Intell Med* A3. https://jmai.amegroups.com/article/view/5930/html.

192 ***Researchers at Penn*** - Stokes, D. C., et al. 2020. "Public Priorities and Concerns Regarding COVID-19 in an Online Discussion Forum: Longitudinal Topic Modeling." *J Gen Intern Med* 35:2244–47.

193 ***Algorithms to read*** - Borkowski, A. A., et al. 2020. "Using Artificial Intelligence for COVID-19 Chest X-ray Diagnosis." *Fed Pract* 37:398–404.

193 ***Scientists from New York*** - Shamout, F. E., et al. 2021. "An Artificial Intelligence System for Predicting the Deterioration of COVID-19 Patients in the Emergency Department." *npj Digit Med* 4:1–11.

193 ***Even vaccine development*** - Wang, J., et al. 2022. "Scaffolding Protein Functional Sites Using Deep Learning." *Science* 377:387–94.

PART IV: MAKING OUR SYSTEM SUSTAINABLE

15: THE VALUE PROPOSITION AND INCENTIVIZING CHANGE

198 ***Volume to value*** - Singh, J. P., and D. J. Wilber. 2015. "Electrophysiology and Health Care Reform: Expanding Our Value Proposition." *JACC: Clin Electrophysiol* 1:463–64.

199 ***Caught in the middle*** - Singh, J. P. 2016. "Resynchronizing the Heart and Remodeling Healthcare." *JACC Clin Electrophysiol* 2:532–33.

199 ***The newer payment schemes*** - Singh, J. P. 2017. "Clinical EP in 2017 and Beyond: Adapting to Payment Reform." *JACC Clin Electrophysiol* 3:85–87.

200 ***Is a moving target*** - 2017. "What Is Value-Based Healthcare?" *NEJM Catalyst*. https://catalyst.nejm.org/doi/full/10.1056/CAT.17.0558.

200 ***Better outcomes that are cost*** - Jain, S. H. 2022. "Everybody's Talking about Value-Based Health Care. Here's What They're Not Saying." *Forbes*. https://www.forbes.com/sites/sachinjain/2022/04/12/what-is-value-based-healthcare-really/.

202 ***In our experience*** - Wasfy, J. H., et al. 2016. "Longer-Term Impact of Cardiology e-Consults." *Am Heart J* 173:86–93.

202 ***My team has recently*** - Zhao, M., et al. 2021. "Virtual Multidisciplinary Care for Heart Failure Patients with Cardiac Resynchronization Therapy Devices during the Coronavirus Disease 2019 Pandemic." *Int J Cardiol Heart Vasc* 34:100811.

203 ***Scrutinized more than 1.5 million*** - Jiang, J., A.-F. Cameron, and M. Yang. 2020. "Analysis of Massive Online Medical Consultation Service Data to Understand Physicians' Economic Return: Observational Data Mining Study." JMIR Med Inform 8 (2):e16765.

203 ***Generating more revenue*** - Butala, N. M., et al. 2019. "Measuring Individual Physician Clinical Productivity in an Era of Consolidated Group Practices." *Healthc (Amst)* 7 (4).

205 ***These are the centerpiece*** - Wenzel, R. P. 2019. "RVU Medicine, Technology, and Physician Loneliness." *N Eng J Med* A380:305–7.

206 ***The fee for each service*** - AAPC. 2022. "What Are Relative Value Ulnites (RVUs)?" https://www.aapc.com/practice-management/rvus.aspx.

206 ***Expense of the physician's*** - Maxwell, S., and S. Zuckerman. 2007. "Impact of Resource-Based Practice Expenses on the Medicare Physician Volume." *Health Care Financ Rev* 29:65–79.

16: CHOOSING THE RIGHT PATH

209 ***His book* The Innovator's Dilemma** - Christensen, C. M. 2011. *The Innovator's Dilemma: The Revolutionary Book That Will Change the Way You Do Business*. New York: HarperBusiness.

211 ***Culture of care*** - Wasfy, J. H., et al. 2020. "Association of an Acute Myocardial Infarction Readmission-Reduction Program With Mortality and Readmission." *Circ Cardiovasc Qual Outcomes* 13:e006043.

211 ***Changing care patterns*** - Musich, S., et al. 2016. "The Impact of Personalized Preven-

tive Care on Health Care Quality, Utilization, and Expenditures." *Popul Health Manag* 19:389–97.

212 ***A study I collaborated*** - Maille, B., et al. 2021. "Smartwatch Electrocardiogram and Artificial Intelligence for Assessing Cardiac-Rhythm Safety of Drug Therapy in the COVID-19 Pandemic. The QT-logs study." *Int J Cardiol* 331:333–39.

213 ***Sensors can predict*** - Gardner, R. S., et al. 2018. "HeartLogic Multisensor Algorithm Identifies Patients during Periods of Significantly Increased Risk of Heart Failure Events: Results from the MultiSENSE Study." *Circ Heart Fail* 11:e004669.

213 ***Sensors can predict*** - Merchant, F. M., G. W. Dec, and J. P. Singh. 2010. "Implantable Sensors for Heart Failure." *Circ Arrhythm Electrophysiol* 3:657–67.

214 ***The quarterback may be*** - Singh, J. P., and D. J. Wilber. 2015. "Electrophysiology and Health Care Reform: Expanding Our Value Proposition." *JACC: Clin Electrophysiol* A1:463–64.

214 ***Health care they receive needs to be valued*** - Porter, M. E. 2010. "What Is Value in Health Care?" *N Engl J Med* A363:2477–81.

216 ***Latin American Telemedicine Infarct Network*** - Mehta, S., et al. 2021. "Impact of a Telemedicine-Guided, Population-Based, STEMI Network on Reperfusion Strategy, Efficiency, and Outcomes." *AsiaIntervention* 7:18–26.

218 ***Helped lead the international*** - Troughton, R. W., et al. 2011. "Direct Left Atrial Pressure Monitoring in Severe Heart Failure: Long-Term Sensor Performance." *J Cardiovasc Transl Res* 4:3–13.

17: FUTURE MODELS OF CARE

222 ***The world of clinical care*** - Singh, J. P. 2021. "Systemness: The Promised Land of Medicine?" *Medscape.* http://www.medscape.com/viewarticle/957918.

223 ***Creates distinct pressure points*** - Willis, D. 2019. "Why Most Systems Struggle with Systemness." *Advisory Board.* https://www.advisory.com/Blog/2019/04/systemness-one.

224 ***The e-patient is educated*** - PatientsLikeMe. 2022. *Wikipedia.*

225 ***In many cases it did not*** - Chatterjee, N. A., and J. P. Singh. 2017. "Making Sense of Remote Monitoring Studies in Heart Failure." *Eur Heart J* 38: 2361–63.

226 ***An array of digital tools*** - Muller, E. "Common Remote Patient Monitoring Devices." *Health Recovery Solutions.* https://www.healthrecoverysolutions.com/blog/7-common-remote-patient-monitoring-devices.

228 ***By 2030, eighty-three million*** - Waters, H., and M. Graf. 2018. "Chronic Diseases Are Taxing Our Health Care System and Our Economy." *STAT.* https://www.statnews.com/2018/05/31/chronic-diseases-taxing-health-care-economy/.

228 ***Shared saving strategies*** - Kapoor, M. 2020. "What Are Shared-Savings Programs?" *Advisory Board.* https://www.advisory.com/Topics/Life-Sciences/2020/05/What-are-shared-savings-programs.

228 ***Patient empowerment*** - Blondon, K., et al. 2014. "An Exploration of Attitudes toward the Use of Patient Incentives to Support Diabetes Self-Management." *Psychol Health* 29:552–63.

229 ***Digital technology from an*** - Zhao, M., J. H. Wasfy, and J. P. Singh. 2020. "Sensor-Aided Continuous Care and Self-Management: Implications for the Post-COVID Era." *Lancet Digit Health* 2:e632–e634.

229 ***If patients are incentivized*** - Kim Farina, P. 2013. "Can Financial Incentives Improve Self-Management Behaviors?" *Evidence-Based Diabetes Management* 19:SP2.

230 ***Prior relationship with a primary care physician*** - Dafny, L. S. 2018. "Does CVS-Aetna Spell the End of Business as Usual?" *N Engl J Med* 378:593–95.

231 ***For example, at Massachusetts General Hospital*** - Martin, L. M., et al. 2018. "Clinical Profile of Acute Myocardial Infarction Patients Included in the Hospital Readmissions Reduction Program." *J Am Heart Assoc* 7:e009339.

233 ***Than the banking industry*** - Christensen, C. M. 2011. *The Innovator's Dilemma: The Revolutionary Book That Will Change the Way You Do Business.* New York: HarperBusiness.

234 ***Andy Ellner*** - Stein, C. 2019. "How an Innovative Partnership Is Helping Firefly Soar." *Blue Cross Blue Shield MA MediaRoom.* https://coverage.bluecrossma.com/.

235 ***The ecosystem*** - Reuter, E. 2021. "Teladoc Backs National Virtual Primary Care Plan for Self-Funded Companies." *MedCity News.* https://medcitynews.com/2021/08/teladoc-backs-national-virtual-primary-care-plan-for-self-funded-companies/.

235 ***The ecosystem is changing*** - Soper, T. 2020. "Virtual Primary Care Startup 98point6 Raises $118M as Pandemic Sparks Demand for Digital Health Tech." *GeekWire.* https://www.geekwire.com/2020/virtual-primary-care-startup-98point6-raises-118m-pandemic-sparks-demand-digital-health-tech/.

235 ***Become a high value soon*** - Norris, L. 2022. "ACA Health Plans Increasingly Offer Wellness Incentives." *healthinsurance.org.* https://www.healthinsurance.org/obamacare/aca-health-plans-increasingly-offer-wellness-incentives/.

236 ***Younger consumers are more likely*** - Kvedar, J. 2022. "Planning for the Next Phase of

Telehealth: Scenarios." https://joekvedar.com/planning-for-the-next-phase-of-telehealth-scenarios/ (2022).

236 ***There is a new generation of*** - Gharib, L., et al. 2021. "Disruptive and Sustaining Innovation in Telemedicine: A Strategic Roadmap." *NEJM Catalyst | Innovations in Care Delivery*. https://catalyst.nejm.org/doi/full/10.1056/CAT.

238 ***It is humbling to*** - Braveman, P., and L. Gottlieb. 2014. "The Social Determinants of Health: It's Time to Consider the Causes of the Causes." *Public Health Rep* 129:19–31.

18: HOSPITAL OF THE FUTURE

247 ***Will reflect not a building*** - Thomas, S. 2022. "The Digital Hospital of the Future." *Deloitte*. https://www2.deloitte.com/global/en/pages/life-sciences-and-healthcare/articles/global-digital-hospital-of-the-future.html.

247 ***Every hospital system*** - "Hospital Command Centers: Urgent Matters." *George Washington University School of Medicine and Health Sciences*. https://smhs.gwu.edu/urgentmatters/news/hospital-command-centers.

248 ***Machine-learning approaches*** - Dawoodbhoy, F. M., et al. 2021. "AI in Patient Flow: Applications of Artificial Intelligence to Improve Patient Flow in NHS Acute Mental Health Inpatient Units." *Heliyon* 7:e06993.

248 ***Alarm fatigue*** - Fernandes, C. O., et al. 2019. "Artificial Intelligence Technologies for Coping with Alarm Fatigue in Hospital Environments Because of Sensory Overload: Algorithm Development and Validation." *J Med Internet Res* 21:e15406.

249 ***Enhancing operational efficiencies*** - Mills, T. 2022. "Council Post: AI For Health And Hope: How Machine Learning Is Being Used In Hospitals." *Forbes*. https://www.forbes.com/sites/forbestechcouncil/2022/02/16/ai-for-health-and-hope-how-machine-learning-is-being-used-in-hospitals/.

251 ***Ambient technology*** - Wigmore, I. "What Is Ambient Intelligence (AmI)?" *SearchEnterpriseAI*. https://www.techtarget.com/searchenterpriseai/definition/ambient-intelligence-AmI.

252 ***Future hospital systems*** - Kumar, S., P. Tiwari, and M. Zymbler. 2019. "Internet of Things Is a Revolutionary Approach for Future Technology Enhancement: A Review." *J Big Data* 6:111. https://doi.org/10.1186/s40537-019-0268-2.

253 ***In their own homes*** - Terry, K. 2020. "CMS Launches Hospital-at-Home Program to Free Up Hospital Capacity." *Medscape*. http://www.medscape.com/viewarticle/941767.

254 ***Practices have begun*** - Klein, S. "'Hospital at Home' Programs Improve Outcomes,

Lower Costs but Face Resistance from Providers and Payers." *Commonwealth Fund.* https://www.commonwealthfund.org/publications/newsletter-article/hospital-home-programs-improve-outcomes-lower-costs-face-resistance.

255 ***Sensor-based approaches*** - Mullaney, T. 2018. "Explosion in Artificial Intelligence Coming for Home Care and Hospitals." *Home Health Care News.* https://homehealthcarenews.com/2018/06/explosion-in-artificial-intelligence-coming-for-home-care-and-hospitals/.

255 ***A few years ago*** - Sainz J. M. 2018. "What the Hospitals of the Future Look Like." *Cirrus Blog.* https://www.getcirrus.com/blog/what-the-hospitals-of-the-future-look-like.

259 ***Symptom checker*** - Isabel Healthcare. 2022. "Isabel—the Symptom Checker Doctors Use and Trust." https://symptomchecker.isabelhealthcare.com.

260 ***The metaverse is an*** - Singh, J. P. 2022. "Meta Medicine: Are We Ready for the Mediverse?" *Medscape.* https://www.medscape.com/viewarticle/978940.

260 ***Mental health*** - Ifdil, I., et al. 2022. "Virtual Reality in Metaverse for Future Mental Health-Helping Profession: An Alternative Solution to the Mental Health Challenges of the COVID-19 Pandemic." *Journal of Public Health.* doi:10.1093/pubmed/fdac049.

260 ***Surgeons to practice*** - Koo, H. 2021. "Training in Lung Cancer Surgery through the Metaverse, Including Extended Reality, in the Smart Operating Room of Seoul National University Bundang Hospital, Korea." *J Educ Eval Health Prof* 18:33. https://www.jeehp.org/DOIx.php?id=10.3352/jeehp.2021.18.33.

261 ***A few years ago*** - "5 Medical Robots Making a Difference in Healthcare at CWRU." 2017. *Case Western Reserve University.* https://online-engineering.case.edu/blog/medical-robots-making-a-difference.

261 ***Cyber knife*** - Shiomi, H., et al. 2001. "Cyber Knife." *Igaku Butsuri* 21:11–16.

261 ***Veebot*** - Perry, T. S. 2013. "Profile: Veebot." *IEEE Spectrum.* https://spectrum.ieee.org/profile-veebot.

261 ***Origami*** - Rus, D., and M. T. Tolley. 2018. "Design, Fabrication and Control of Origami Robots." *Nat Rev Mater* 3:101–12.

261 ***Pharma-assist robots*** - Kent, C. 2021. "Drug Dispensing Goes Digital." *Pharmaceutical Technology.* https://www.pharmaceutical-technology.com/analysis/robotic-drug-dispensing-digital-pharmacy/.

262 ***XDBOT*** - "NTU Builds Disinfection Robot to Tackle COVID-19 Outbreak." 2020. *BioSpectrum.* https://www.biospectrumasia.com/news/54/15807/ntu-builds-disinfection-robot-to-tackle-covid-19-outbreak.html.

263 ***Robots will fill this shortage*** - Diaz, N. 2022. "Hospital Robots Bolstering Nurses

Energy, Time." *Becker's Health IT.* https://www.beckershospitalreview.com/healthcare-information-technology/hospital-robots-bolstering-nurses-energy-time.html.

263 ***Nearly 50 percent*** - Kelly, J. 2022. "New Survey Shows That Up to 47% of U.S. Healthcare Workers Plan to Leave Their Positions by 2025." *Forbes.* https://www.forbes.com/sites/jackkelly/2022/04/19/new-survey-shows-that-up-to-47-of-us-healthcare-workers-plan-to-leave-their-positions-by-2025/.

263 ***Global shortage*** - World Health Organization. 2013. "Global Health Workforce Shortage to Reach 12.9 Million in Coming Decades." https://apps.who.int/mediacentre/news/releases/2013/health-workforce-shortage/en/index.html.

INDEX